Essentials of Exercise Physiology

Essentials of Exercise Physiology

Shyamal Koley PhD

Head and Dean
Faculty of Sports Medicine and Physiotherapy
Guru Nanak Dev University
Amritsar, Punjab, India

Foreword
GL Khanna

JAYPEE

JAYPEE BROTHERS MEDICAL PUBLISHERS
The Health Sciences Publisher
New Delhi | London

Jaypee Brothers Medical Publishers (P) Ltd

Headquarters
EMCA House
23/23-B, Ansari Road, Daryaganj
New Delhi 110 002, India
Landline: +91-11-23272143,
+91-11-23272703
+91-11-23282021, +91-11-23245672
E-mail: jaypee@jaypeebrothers.com

Corporate Office
Jaypee Brothers Medical Publishers (P) Ltd.
4838/24, Ansari Road, Daryaganj
New Delhi 110 002, India
Phone: +91-11-43574357
Fax: +91-11-43574314
E-mail: jaypee@jaypeebrothers.com

Overseas Office
JP Medical Ltd.
83, Victoria Street, London
SW1H 0HW (UK)
Phone: +44-20 3170 8910
E-mail: info@jpmedpub.com

EU GPSR Authorised Representative
Logos Europe, 9 rue Nicolas Poussin
17000, La Rochelle, France
Phone: +33 (0) 6 67 93 73 78
E-mail: Contact@logoseurope.eu

Website: www.jaypeebrothers.com
Website: www.jaypeedigital.com

Essentials of Exercise Physiology

First Edition: 2018, Reprint: **2025**

ISBN: 978-93-5270-509-2

Printed in India

Dedicated to

My Teachers, Mentors and
my beloved Students

Foreword

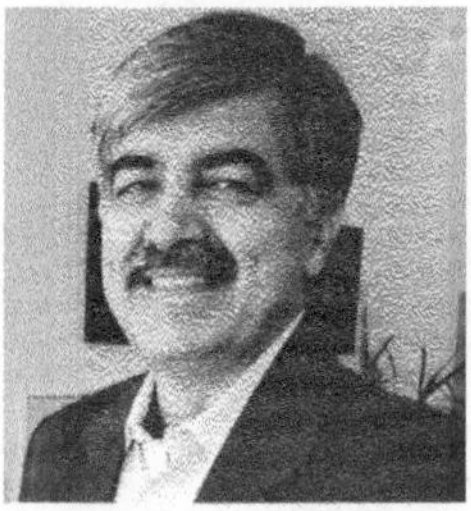

It is my immense pleasure and proud privilege to write the foreword for *Essentials of Exercise Physiology* by Shyamal Koley.

Exercise physiology is an important aspect of Sports Medicine, Sports Physiotherapy, Sports Sciences, Physical Education and many other allied fields. Most of the books available for this subject are written by overseas authors. However, books from Indian authors are scanty in this regard. Most of the books are voluminous also which draw less interest to the general students towards the subject. This book is very concise and written in a very simple and easy language which the students will feel handy.

This book is a great boon for the undergraduate and postgraduate students, researchers and teachers for easy references. I strongly appreciate the author for his boldness to bring this book. I pray to the almighty for the success of Prof Koley in this endeavor.

GL Khanna
Dean, Faculty of Applied Sciences
Director, Manav Rachna Sports Science Centre
Manav Rachna International University
Faridabad, Haryana
President, Asian Council of Exercise and Sports Sciences
Member, Olympic Task Force, India

Preface

Exercise physiology is an essential aspect of Sports Medicine which deals with the biological explanations of human body functioning on the light of exercise. This subject is getting tremendous importance from every corner of the globe for its applied value. The book is written on the applied aspects of Exercise Physiology, making it very concise and simple, especially for the UG and PG students of Sports Medicine, Sports Physiotherapy, Physical Education, Sports Sciences, Physical Anthropology, Human Biology, and many other allied fields. Researchers and teachers of these fields will also be benefited greatly in updating their recent knowledge from this book. The book deals with 14 chapters containing effects of exercise on various systems of our body which are discussed in a very simple manner and written in a very lucid language. Books in the field of applied exercise physiology by Indian authors are scanty, thus the book is planned by incorporating all the important aspects of applied exercise physiology.

Shyamal Koley

Acknowledgments

I take the opportunity to express my gratitude to all those who were instrumental to prepare the manuscript. I am thankful to Prof GL Khanna, Dean, Faculty of Applied Science and Director, Manav Rachna Sports Science Centre, Manav Rachna International University, Faridabad, Haryana, India, for his constant inspiration, support and encouragement to go ahead with the thoughts of writing the book and also for writing the foreword of this book.

I am also thankful to my postgraduate students, especially Nihar Ranjan Mohanty, Avinash Tiwari and Davinder Singh for their cooperation. I would be failing in my duties if I do not acknowledge my thanks to my colleagues who extended their support to write the book. I am thankful to Mr Arun Bajaj, Office Superintendent of the department for computation of the manuscript.

Thanks are also due to my publisher M/s Jaypee Brothers Medical Publishers (P) Ltd, New Delhi, for making efforts in bringing out this book.

Last but not least, I would like to express my thanks to my family, wife Kakali Koley, daughters Gagari and Hiya, and son Raunak for their constant support to prepare this manuscript.

Contents

CHAPTER 1

Introduction

The term physiology was derived from the Greek word 'Physiologikos' meaning discourse on natural knowledge. Physiology deals with the normal functioning of human body. Studies of physiology have some branches, viz. viral physiology, bacterial physiology, cell physiology, plant physiology, animal physiology, human physiology, etc. Human physiology may further be divided into exercise physiology, nutritional physiology, etc. In this volume, only the contents of exercise physiology will be discussed.

In dictionary, health is defined as freedom from disease. A more searching look into this subject would show that health is more than this. In ancient Greek literature, health had not been considered as a single entity. They used two separate words, viz. heuexia and hygieia. Heuexia means a good habit of body and hygieia is a good way of living. They also knew the close association of mind and body. So, we should establish good habits of living for the well-being of our body.

According to World Health Organization (WHO) health is a state of complete physical, mental and social well-being and not merely the absence of disease and infirmity. It is difficult to quantify health in this positive sense. Nevertheless, negative indices like illness, disability, mortality rates are also taken into account by physicians to assess the health.

Nowadays, we are passing through such an environmental phase where we are simply encountering with pollutants in every moment. Urbanization and industrialization bring comfort and affluence; make our lives pleasant, jubilant and luxuriant. At the same time they render numerous complications and diseases. For instance, we may consider only a single complication—obesity. Researchers inform that obese people are often hypertensive and have elevated serum lipid levels. Mechanical disabilities like flat feet, osteoarthritis of knee, hip, lumbar spine, abdominal hernias, diaphragmatic hernias, varicose veins, respiratory infections are associated with obesity. The health risks of obesity also include autonomic and ventricular dysfunction, adult onset diabetes mellitus, renal diseases, problems in administering anesthetics during surgery, several types of cancer, menstrual irregularities and enormous psychological burden.

Exercise physiology is the scientific study of physiological changes in athletes' body with the effects of exercise, whether long term or short term. Different environmental changes, viz. altitude, climate, temperature, humidity, nutritional status, etc. have some close associations with the optimal performance of an athlete. The objectives of the exercise physiologists are to assess the working capacity and to examine the physical fitness of the athletes. The other important aspects of studying the exercise physiology are to enhance the physical performance of the athletes to its peak and to keep the injuries at bay. Success is the main goal of all sports persons in any international competition. For optimal performances, most athletes have the interest in optimizing their total physiological capacity for their respective sports events.

Apart from these, health status, drugs, sleep, anxiety, etc. also affect the performance of athletes. Therefore, good health, good habits, good way of living and sound techniques of various sports events are the main *mantras* for the success of any sports. Knowledge of exercise physiology makes an athlete well-equipped to participate in competitive sports.

FITNESS

Fitness is essentially a matter of the amount of exercise an individual can tolerate. The concept of exercise tolerance is important as a way of assessing heart and lung diseases. This exercise tolerance scale exhibits the fitness hierarchy where marathoners are at the top and bedridden heart patients are at the bottom. Fitness may be measured in terms of travelled distance by brisk walking till breathlessness compels them to stop. Majority of people has low fitness level with sedentary lifestyle and minimum physical activities. People with low fitness level but free from diseases surely can increase their tolerance levels, irrespective to age, sex, profession, etc. by doing regular physical exercise. Sports persons are directly involved in regular physical exercise to enhance their performances in competitions of different levels.

BENEFITS OF EXERCISE

Exercise has enormous beneficial effects in our body. Physiologically, it benefits virtually every system and cell of the body. Some of those are given as follows:

- It increases the size of the muscle fibers, consequently increasing the muscle mass and muscular activity in the body.
- It increases bone calcium, thus helps in maintenance of bone mass, particularly in the later age and postmenopausal women.
- It increases cardiac output, increasing the stroke volume of the heart. It produces electric stability of the heart muscles reducing the risk of cardiac arrhythmia.
- It increases venous return.
- It increases hemoglobin concentration in the blood, providing better oxygen carrying capacity.
- It increases vascular resistance in the inactive muscles.
- It inhibits the blood clotting process and stickiness of the blood, contributing reduction in heart attacks.
- It increases oxygen pick up in the lungs.
- It increases oxygen supply in the heart, muscles and increases greater extraction of oxygen at the peripheral level.
- It strengthens the tendons, ligaments, muscles and other tissues around the joints, lubricating the joint cartilages and capsules, maintaining proper flexibility of joints. Greater the flexibility of joints, lesser will be the chances of injury.
- It decreases resting heart rate.
- It avoids senility – increases oxygen delivery of brain.
- It activates the sympathetic nervous system and puts the whole body on the alert.
- It increases gastrointestinal tone.
- It lowers the blood cholesterol which is a major risk factor in coronary heart disease, improving blood high density cholesterol (HDL), which is cardioprotective.
- It decreases blood triglycerides.
- Blood pressure increases during exercise, but in the long run, it decreases the blood pressure.

- It decreases insulin requirement, increases insulin-sensitivity, thus ameliorates diabetes mellitus.
- It increases glycogen storage.
- It burns carbohydrate (sugar), thus helps in less conversion of sugar to fat.
- It helps better control of hunger, increasing the level of leptin in the circulation.
- It decreases body fat. It benefits the cardiovascular system by reducing body weight.
- It enhances metabolic functions by controlling the body weight, thus preventing obesity.
- It increases aerobic threshold.
- It decreases stress (attitude).
- It increases ability to handle stress (biochemical).
- It improves resistance to cold.
- It increases basal metabolic rate (BMR).
- It decreases load on the heart.
- It decreases muscle dependence on sugar.
- It increases emotional lift.
- It helps in increased production of endorphine by the brain which is nature's own opiates.
- The physical exercise has positive influence on the psychological functioning also. It reduces anxiety and depression, thus elevates the mood.
- It enhances the psychomotor development and capacity to face impediments.
- It improves memory and increases self-esteem.

In the present volume, the effects of exercise on all the important systems of human body are discussed in a very concise manner. The systems include:

- Skeletal system—dealing with bones and joints
- Muscular system—dealing with skeletal muscles only
- Cardiovascular system—dealing with the heart and blood vessels
- Respiratory system—dealing with lungs
- Endocrine system—dealing with various endocrine glands and their hormones
- Nervous system—dealing with the nerves and their controls
- Digestive system—dealing with ingestion and metabolism of foods

- Excretory system—dealing with renal function
- Reproductive system—dealing with the functions of sex hormones.

Apart from these systems, the present volume deals with:

- Nutrition
- Temperature regulation
- Gender differences on physical performances
- Manipulation of body composition status in athletes.

CHAPTER 2

Effects of Exercise on Skeletal System

The skeleton is a living, dynamic system in our body. The bony and cartilaginous framework of the human body constitutes the skeleton. It is of two types—endoskeleton and exoskeleton. In endoskeleton, the skeleton is confined within the body. In humans, the term skeleton means endoskeleton. Exoskeleton is very rudimentary, represented by nails and enamel of the teeth only. The condition of bone is improved by exercise, because it responds to mechanical stresses. The mechanical stresses regulate bone size and structure in combination with nutritional status, genetic set-up and biochemical reactions (Carton, 1987; Frost, 1990; Cowin, 1991 and Lanyon, 1992). The mechanical stresses generally act in the form of skeletal muscle pulling at their points of attachment, i.e. origins and insertions. It has been reported that more mineral salts are deposited and more collagenous fibers are produced where these mechanical stresses are applied most. Therefore, in these areas, both the density and size of bone increase. These changes in bone structure are stimulated by increased loads exerted on the skeleton. Bone adaptation to exercise is a slow process; therefore, the increments in size and strength are also slower, resulting measurements of bone adaptation difficult. The anterior and posterior views of human skeleton are shown in Figures 2.1 and 2.2.

COMPOSITION OF BONE

Water—25%
Solid—75%.
Of the solids, following substances are present:

- Proteinous organic substances—30%
  - Scleroprotein named ossein
  - Mucoprotein named osseomucoid
  - Ceratinoprotein named osseoalbumin

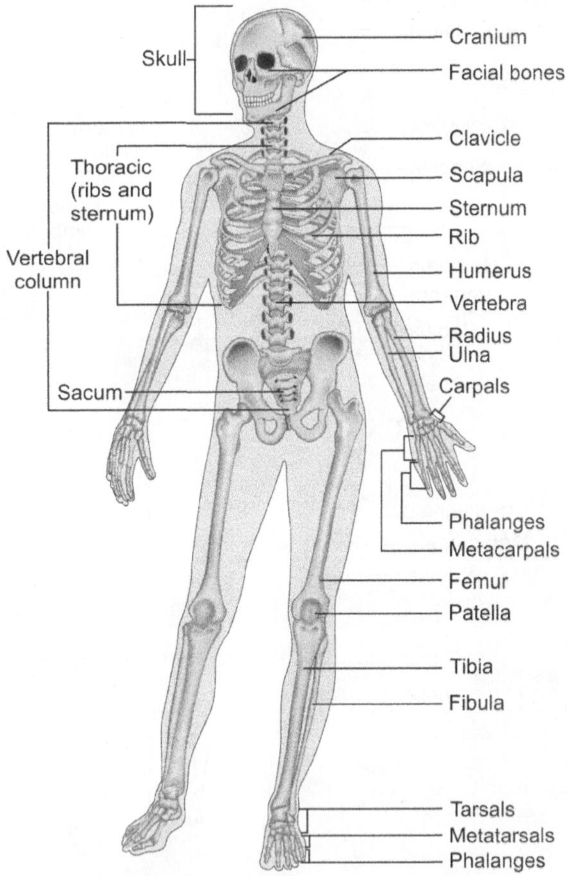

Fig. 2.1: Anterior view of human skeleton

These proteinous organic substances are responsible for toughness and resilience of bone.

- Inorganic substances - 45%
  - Calcium phosphate - 3.6%
  - Calcium carbonate - 5.8%
  - Magnesium phosphate - 0.9%
  - Calcium chloride } - 2.3%
  - Calcium fluoride }

These inorganic substances are responsible for the rigidity and hardness of bone. The presence of calcium makes the bone opaque to X-ray.

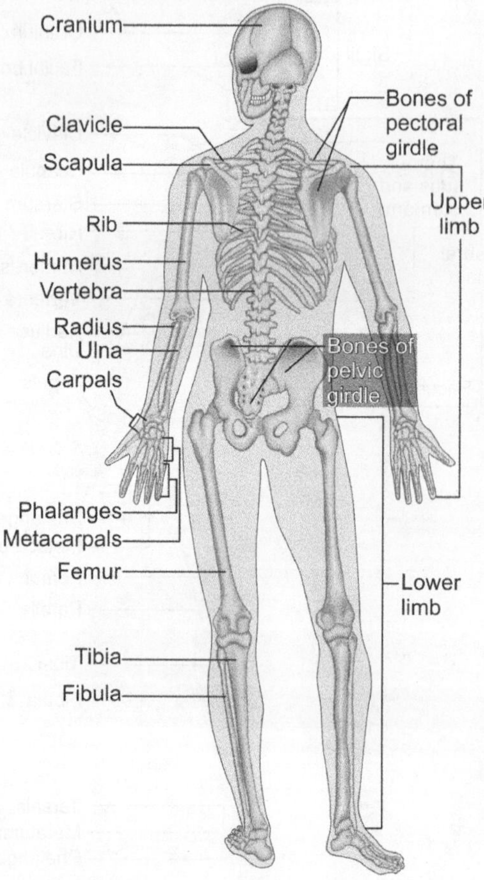

Fig. 2.2: Posterior view of human skeleton

Functions of Bones

- Bones and cartilages which make up the skeleton are the only rigid materials in the body. Bone constitutes the framework of the body giving a specific form to it.
- It forms the central axis of the body.
- It bears the weight of the body.
- Forming articulations and giving attachment to muscles, it provides the levers essential for movement and locomotion. The joints allow movement between bones and these movements are directly related to the types of joint and range of motion.

- It provides mechanical protection to vital organs. Typical examples are skull protects the brain, vertebrae protect the spinal cord, thoracic cage protects the heart and lungs.
- It also serves as a detoxicating agent. Toxic substances, viz. lead, fluorine, arsenic, radium, etc. are removed from the circulation and are deposited in the bones and teeth.
- In some bones, there is red marrow which produces red blood cells, some white cells and platelets.
- It acts as storehouse of calcium in the body. Minerals, especially calcium and phosphorus are stored in bones and can be distributed to other parts of the body.

BONE CELLS (FIG. 2.3)

The cells responsible for the formation of bone are osteoblasts (later develop into osteocytes). Osteoblasts are present in the deeper layers of periosteum, in the centers of ossification of immature bone, at the ends of the diaphysis adjacent to the epiphyseal cartilages of long bones and at the site of fracture.

At the later stage of development, osteoblasts become trapped and remain isolated in lacunae. At this stage, they stop forming new bones and are called osteocytes. Lymph in the canaliculi nourishes the osteocytes. They help in the movement of calcium between bones and the blood.

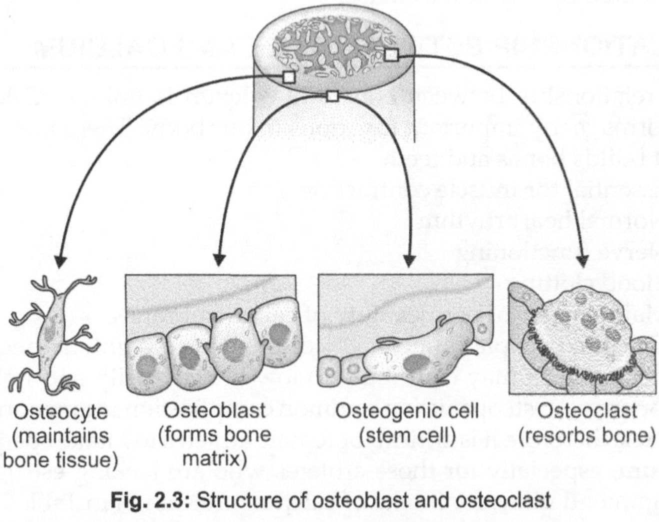

Fig. 2.3: Structure of osteoblast and osteoclast

Osteoclasts are involved in the resorption of bone and by this process, they maintain the optimum shape. Resorption takes place at bone surfaces under the periosteum, to maintain the shape of bones during growth and to remove excess callus formed during healing of fractures.

GROWTH OF BONES

Some hormones regulate the growth and consistency of size and the shape of bones. These are:

- Growth hormone and the thyroid hormones, thyroxine and triiodothyronine are important during infancy and childhood. Growth hormone stimulates the liver to secrete somatomedin. It is a polypeptide with the molecular weight of 7500. Growth hormone increases the synthesis and deposition of proteins chondrocytes and osteogenic cells. Deficiency or excessive secretion of these hormones results abnormal development of the skeleton.
- Testosterone and estrogens responsible for the physical changes in puberty. For example, the growth spurt and masculinizing or feminizing changes of specific parts of the skeleton viz. pelvis.
- Calcitonin from the thyroid gland and parathormone from the parathyroid glands influence in maintaining the calcium levels essential for bone development.

The secretions of all the above-mentioned hormones are stimulated by physical exercise.

RELATIONSHIP BETWEEN BONE AND CALCIUM

The relationship between bone and calcium is unique. Calcium performs many important functions in our body. These are:

- It builds bones and teeth
- Essential for muscle contraction
- Normal heart rhythm
- Nerve functioning
- Blood clotting
- Maintenance of permeability of cell membranes.

Calcium occupies almost 50% of the bone weight. Inadequate dietary calcium may contribute to low bone density and risk for osteoporosis. Osteopenia is a common complication in amenorrheic athletes, therefore it is critical for female athletes to intake adequate calcium, especially for those athletes who are lacking estrogens. Recommendations for intake of calcium are shown in Table 2.1.

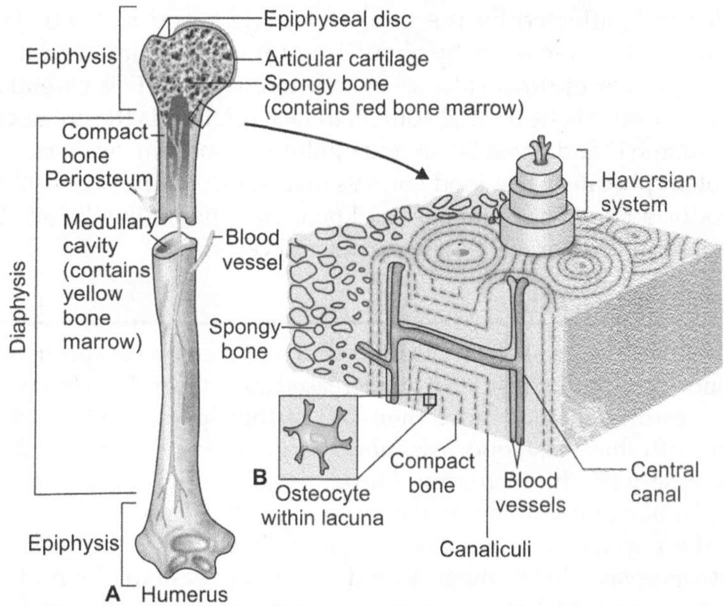

Figs 2.4A and B: Structure of bones

Source: www.slideshare.net/LawrenceJames/histo-bone

Table 2.1: Recommendations for calcium intake (NIH, 1998)

Category	Ages (years)	Calcium intake (mg/day)
Children and young adults	11–24	1200–1500
Premenopausal women	25–50	1000
Pregnant women		Age specific value + 400
Postmenopausal women taking estrogen	Less than 65	1000
Postmenopausal women not taking estrogen	Less than 65	1500
Men	Less than 65	1000
Men and women	65 and above	1500

The amount of parathyroid hormone (PTH) increases in the circulation with the decrease of concentration of ionized calcium in the extracellular fluid. Parathyroid hormone stimulates formation of new osteoclasts and thus enhances bone resorption. Renal tubular calcium reabsorption is also increased by parathyroid hormone reducing urinary calcium loss. The individual requirement of calcium is affected by the intake of protein and salt too. The urine calcium increases by about 1mg for every gram of protein ingested. For optimal calcium absorption, vitamin D is essential. Sun exposure is its natural source. In fact, calcium is the enhancer of vitamin D and phosphorus and inhibitor of sodium, oxalates and protein phylates. The food sources of calcium are milk and milk products (curd, channa, cheese, khoa, etc.), fish, gingelly seeds, ragi, nuts, dark green leaves, pulses and cereals.

OSTEOPOROSIS

Osteoporosis is a skeletal disorder characterized by compromised bone strength that results in an increased susceptibility to fracture. It is estimated that more than 200 million people worldwide currently have osteoporosis, and the prevalence is expected to increase with the increasing lifespan and ageing population. In the United States alone, an estimated 44 million individuals (55% of the population older than 50 years) have low bone mass or osteoporosis. This number is predicted to increase to 61.4 million by the year 2020. Because osteoporosis is seen mainly as a disease that affects women, men often go undiagnosed and untreated, yet men are increasingly at risk for osteoporotic fractures. The clinical relevance of osteoporosis is the dramatic increase in risk of fracture. More than 1.5 million fractures are associated with osteoporosis each year.

Skeletal Fragility

Many skeletal characteristics contribute to bone strength, and consequently, bone fragility, including the quantity of bone material present, the quality of the material, and the distribution of the material within the bone structure.

Bone quantity: Bone 'quantity' refers to the amount of bone material present (i.e. the bone mass). The actual pattern of bone change is more dynamic than shown, both during growth and in later life. Overall, global bone formation continues at a faster pace than bone resorption until peak bone mineral accretion is attained sometime in the second or third decade (depending on site, region, and gender). In later life, the process of bone formation in each remodeling site no longer equals the bone that was resorbed, and thus, a small amount of bone is lost with each new remodeling cycle. This is referred to as a negative bone balance. In later life, gonadal hormones (testosterone, estrogen) decrease in both men and women. Estrogen suppresses activation of new remodeling cycles, and thus, low estrogen levels partially contribute to an increased rate of remodeling. As resorption precedes formation in the process of remodeling, and formation and subsequent mineralization are time-intensive processes, an increase in the rate of remodeling results in temporary decreases in bone mass. Although temporary losses in bone mass lead to a transient increase in bone fragility, increased rates of remodeling with a negative bone balance lead to sustained bone loss of approximately 9 to 13% during the first 5 years after menopause. Bone turnover eventually slows to a rate similar to premenopausal years. Men also experience age-related bone loss but without the rapid period of loss.

Lifestyle modifications: Because of difficulty in implementing long-term lifestyle changes, the exercise professional can play a large role in facilitating adherence to these changes in the patient with osteoporosis.

All postmenopausal women and older men, regardless of fracture risk, should be encouraged to engage in behavior modifications, including adequate calcium (1000–1500 mg per day) and vitamin D (400–800 ID per day) intake, regular exercise, smoking cessation, avoidance of excessive alcohol intake, and visual correction to decrease fall risk. Of these lifestyle modifications, exercise is the only one that can simultaneously ameliorate low BMD, augment muscle mass, promote strength gain, and improve dynamic balance—all of which are independent risk factors for fracture.

Acute Physiological Response

Bone is a dynamic tissue capable of continually adapt to its changing mechanical environment. When a bone is loaded in compression, tension, or torsion, bone tissue is deformed. Deformation of bone tissue, or the relative change in bone length, is referred to as strain.

Bone tissue strain causes fluid within the bone to move past the cell membrane of osteocytes—the bone cells that are embedded throughout bone tissue and are connected with one another, to other bone cells, and with the bone marrow through slender dendritic processes. The current prevailing theory in the bone field is that this fluid flow along the osteocyte and its cell processes causes a release of molecular signals that lead to osteoclast and osteoblast recruitment to (re)model bone to better suit its new mechanical environment. This process of turning a mechanical signal into a biochemical one is called mechanotransduction.

Chronic Physiological Response

- It has been suggested by Harold Frost that the response of bone to its mechanical environment is controlled by a 'mechanostat' that aims to keep bone tissue strain at an optimal level by homeostatically altering bone structure. Indeed, when bone is subjected to lower than customary loads (as in space flight and immobilization), bone will adapt by ridding itself of excess mass.
- Alternately, when bone is subjected to higher loads such as uncustomary exercise, bone will become stronger by altering its structure and increasing in mass. Although mechanotransduction is an acute response to exercise, the adaptation of bone structure through modeling and remodeling takes up to several months to complete.
- Remodeling is a process that not only performs the task of removing excess bone or adding bone on trabecular surfaces in youth but also repairs fatigue-damaged bone. With the increase in bone tissue strain that occurs with exercise, damage in the form of microcracks results. This damage is targeted for removal by osteoclasts, and new bone is formed in its place. Thus, one of the chronic effects of exercise on the skeleton involves the maintenance of bone strength through targeted remodeling.
- Mineralization of newly formed bone is an ongoing process on the order of months to years. Resorption precedes formation in remodeling; therefore, the effects of exercise on the skeleton may take up to several months to be fully realized.

Exercise Prescription in Patients with Osteoporosis

- Prior to prescribing exercise for the patient with osteoporosis, an exercise professional should consult with the clients' physician.
- For patients with debilitating osteoporosis and severe pain or recent joint replacement, exercise program options will be limited. These patients should typically work with a physical therapist or rehabilitation specialist until mobile. There is a high prevalence of back pain in patients with osteoporosis, which is related to limited functional ability.

- Thus, pain management may be an important part of the care for osteoporotic individuals. It may be necessary to begin exercise prescription with a warm-pool-based program (e.g. hydrotherapy), which, although non-weight-bearing, can improve flexibility and muscle strength.
- In light of the rapid and profound effects of immobilization and bed rest on bone loss, and the poor prognosis for recovery of bone mineral content after remobilization, even the frailest elderly people should remain as physically active as their health permits to preserve skeletal integrity.
- If a person cannot tolerate active exercises, functional electrical stimulation may improve vital muscle strength in preparation for active strengthening as pain diminishes.
- As stated in the ACSM position stand on physical activity and bone health, 'exercise programs for elderly women and men should include not only weight-bearing endurance and resistance activities aimed at preserving bone mass, but also activities designed to improve balance and prevent falls.'
- A 20-week strength, posture, and balance program, *Osteofit*, improved dynamic balance in females with osteoporosis.
- In a study of females with a history of spinal fracture, a 10-week balance, strengthening, stretching, and relaxation program resulted in a significant reduction in pain and use of analgesia and increased quality of life.
- In both men and women with osteoporosis, 12 months of balance and strength training resulted in improved BMD, balance, and aerobic capacity.
- Although these trials indicate that exercise has beneficial effects on *surrogates* of osteoporotic fracture, well-designed studies with fracture endpoints are needed to further guide exercise prescription in men and women with osteoporosis.

Contraindicated Exercises for Individuals with Osteoporosis

Several general types of exercise are contraindicated for people with osteoporosis because they can generate large forces on relatively weak bone.

- Twisting movements (e.g. golf swing), dynamic abdominal exercises (e.g. sit-ups), and excessive trunk flexion should all be avoided because they can all result in vertebral fracture.

- Osteoporotic individuals should be taught correct form of ADLs such as bending to pick up objects to avoid vertebral fractures.
- Furthermore, exercises that involve abrupt or explosive loading, or high-impact loading, are contraindicated in persons with osteoporosis.

STRAIN AS A STIMULUS FOR BONE ADAPTATION

The skeleton is a living dynamic system. It adapts to the mechanical loads of exercise. In combination with genetics, nutrition and biochemistry, mechanical forces regulate bone size and structure. It has been observed that bone adaptation to exercise is slower and the increments in size and strength are smaller as compared to other systems. Therefore, measurement of bone adaptation is rather difficult. Nowadays, different exercises which benefit the bone health are widely practiced. Exercise is being recommended even for the prevention of osteoporosis.

One of the functions of bone in our body is to serve as stiff levers and beams for support and movement. Forces generated from muscle contraction and impact loading create compression, tension, torsion and shear stresses within bone, resulting minuscule shape distortions, bending or deformation. During loading, the degree of distortion or strain magnitude is directly proportional to the applied forces and inversely proportional to the size and distribution of the bone. The distribution of bone tissue relative to a neutral axis is measured by moment of inertia (MI) which reflects the resistance of bone to bending. The greater the bone mass and further the mass is located from the neutral axis, the greater would be the moment of inertia and the lower the strain for any given force.

EXERCISE RESPONSE IN BONE

The magnitude of the bone response to mechanical forces depends on the forces and strains created during exercise. Apart from this, hormonal influence, dietary intake, genetic potential and age are also contributing factors included in this direction.

GENETIC POTENTIAL AND EXERCISE

Bone gain with exercise is now a widely accepted concept. The variation in response to exercise ranges from +4 to -2% in college age women and from +15 to -7% in postmenopausal women. Some variations are associated with individual potential for either exercise or bone gain. Johnston and Slemenda (1993) are of the opinion that genetic factors have been associated with 60 to 80% of the variance in bone mass. The potential for bone mass accretion with exercise may be regulated genetically. Moderate correlation between bone mineral content (BMC) and bone mineral density (BMD); and body weight, height and body composition have been observed in some cross sectional studies. These correlations potentially reflect the genetic regulation of musculoskeletal adaptation during exercise.

PHYSICAL ACTIVITY AND BONE ACROSS THE LIFESPAN

The potential effectiveness of exercise to alter the bone mass is affected with factors like developmental age and hormone. Bone modeling is rapid in the growing child, increasing size of the bone. Resorption also helps in shaping the bone. Recker et al. (1992) reported that by the end of third decade of life, peak bone mass would be achieved. In adults, remodeling process continues but bone mass remains stable. In old age, 5% bone loss per decade were reported by Heaney (1990) may be due to remodeling imbalance between resorption and formation. At menopause, with lack of estrogen this imbalance may cause 10 to 15% bone loss within 10 years. Exercise has been proved to modulate each of these development phases.

GROWTH AND PEAK BONE MASS

In early life, the skeletal size is determined by genetic and early developmental factors. Cooper et al. (1995) obtained that body weight at 1 year and height at 5 years are the best predictors of total body bone mineral content in college age adults. The body weight to bone mineral content ratio remains constant with growth. It has been reported that exercise sometimes become a good predictor of bone mineral density (Welten et al. 1994; Ruiz et al., 1995 and Boot et al. 1997). Nonetheless, during growth the most consistent and the stronger predictors have been found as the weight and the Tanner stage.

The exercises of high impact and weight bearing activities have greatest association with bone size in childhood. Slemenda et al. (1991) showed a positive relationship between bone mineral density and current weight bearing activity. Bone mass is found to be greater in competitive weight lifters and gymnasts than controls.

In prepubescent girls, Morris et al. (1997) found that aerobic weight bearing exercise did increase the bone mineral density 2 to 10% more than normal growing control. Likewise, 1 year elite gymnasts were reported to have 32 to 85% greater gain in bone mineral density than controls. In the findings of Forwood and Parker (1987), gymnasts' bones tended to be shorter and thicker than controls, but having greater density may be due to strenuous exercise in growing stages. Albeit, strenuous exercise may suppress longitudinal growth.

If greater physical activity is started before puberty and continues up to college days, the chances would be maximum to have greatest potential for increasing bone mass. Kannus et al. (1995) reported that prepubertal training in tennis, gymnastics and ballet was associated with greater adult bone mineral content. In fact, peak bone mass is achieved by the late 20's. Recker et al. (1992) stated that physical activity during that period had a positive impact on bone mass.

APPROPRIATE EXERCISE

Low intensity exercises have very little impact in bone gain because they create very little strain on bone. Instead, high intensity exercises like gymnastics generate high and varied forces at multiple angles and frequencies to create optimal strains on bone. Therefore, these high intensity exercises are most effective in bone gain. Research findings show that athletes in racket sports, basketball, volleyball, dance and weight lifting, get advantages to gain in lumbar and femoral bone mass.

For maximizing bone mass and maintaining it throughout life, the most effective recommendations are of four fold:

- The metabolic conditions must be optimized like proper balance of calcium through adequate nutrition.
- Exercise must stress the targeted bones exerting adequate force, repetitions and varied movements.
- Start moving and playing from the early stages of life and continue it throughout, have maximum fun and fitness.
- Sedentary people should not think that it is too late to start or restart an exercise program. Start exercise at any stage of life.

CHAPTER 3

Effects of Exercise on Muscular System

Muscle is the contractile tissue of our body. It has four main properties, viz.

1. Excitability – ability to respond to stimuli.
2. Contractibility – ability to contract.
3. Extensibility – ability of a muscle to be stretched without tearing.
4. Elasticity – ability to return to its normal shape.

These unique properties of skeletal muscle are highly susceptible to adaptive changes. This plasticity is manifested by its changes induced by exercise or altered activity. Some of the important factors to be considered in examining skeletal muscle adaptations are:

- The nuclei are postmitotic.
- The cells are multinucleated, consisting of several hundred to several thousand nuclei per centimeter length of a fiber.
- Different isoforms of structural proteins and enzymes are manifested.
- Space constraints within a fiber limit the noncontractile components (mitochondria, lipids, and other sarcoplasmic contents), so muscle fibers must maximize the use of the space available to them.

CLASSIFICATION

Structurally, there are three types of muscle tissue. These are:

1. Striated, skeletal or voluntary muscle
2. Nonstriated, involuntary, visceral or smooth muscle
3. Cardiac muscle.

COMPOSITION OF SKELETAL MUSCLES

- Water—75%
- Solid—25%

- Proteins—20%, actin and myosin occupy about 50% of the total muscle proteins.
- Fats—0.2%, including neutral fat, cholesterol and lecithin.
- Carbohydrates—1.0%, glycogen—0.5 to 1.0%, hexose phosphate —0.05%.
- Inorganic salts—1.0—1.5%, potassium phosphate—0.3%, traces of calcium (0.007%), sodium (0.06%), magnesium (0.02%), iron, chlorine, sulfate, phosphates remain in various forms (0.06%).
- Extractives: Non-nitrogenous
- Lactic acid—0.02% (in fresh resting muscle)
- Inositol—0.25% nitrogenous
- Adenosine triphosphate (ATP)—0.25%
- Adenosine diphosphate (ADP)—0.1%
- Adenosine monophosphate (AMP)—0.15%
- Creatine phosphate—Phosphocreatine or phosphagen—0.5% (creatine—0.35%).
- Xanthine, hypoxanthine and inosinic acid—derived from adenylic acid of the tissue and the nucleoprotein of the nuclei.
- Carnosine—0.3%
- Pigments:
  - Myoglobin
  - Cytochrome
  - Flavines and others.
- Enzymes and coenzymes:
  - Enzymes and coenzymes of the glycolytic cycle.
  - Those that breakdown and resynthesize ATP and phosphagen.
  - Enzymes of the citric acid cycle, that finally oxidize pyruvic acid into CO_2 and H_2O.
  - Other enzymes like deaminase, etc.

FUNCTIONS OF SKELETAL MUSCLE

The muscular system performs three important functions. These are:

1. Motion—walking, running, etc.
2. Heat production—maintain normal body temperature.
3. Maintenance of posture—standing, sitting, etc.

Motion

The muscles combine with the skeleton and provide the motion. We know that the main framework of the body is covered by muscles and permits movement. In the principle of physics, levers are used to move or lift a load against another force. We also adapt the same principle in our musculoskeletal system. The component parts which are used in a lever are as follows:

- Lever – nearly always the bone shaft.
- Fulcrum – pivot point of the lever which is usually the joint.
- Muscle force – force that draws the opposite ends of the muscle together.
- Resistive force – force generated by factors external to the body (e.g. gravity, friction, etc.) and internal like ligamentous and capsular tension that acts against muscle force.
- Torque – the degree to which a force tends to rotate an object about a specified fulcrum.

Depending upon the position of fulcrum, effort and resistive force, the lever may be classified into three classes:

1. First class lever: In this case muscle force and resistive force are on different sides of the fulcrum, e.g. the head resting on the vertebral column. As the head is raised, the facial portion of the skull is the resistance, the fulcrum is between the atlas and occipital bone, and the effort is the contraction of the muscles of the back.
2. Second class lever: In this case, muscle force and resistance force act on the same side of the fulcrum, with the muscle force acting through the level longer than that through which the resistive force acts, e.g. rising the body up onto the toes. The body is the resistance, the ball of the foot is the fulcrum, and the effort is the contraction of the calf muscle.
3. Third class lever: In this case, muscle force and resistive force act on the same side of the fulcrum, with the muscle force acting through the lever shorter than that through which the resistive force acts, e.g. adduction of the thigh. The weight of the thigh is the resistance, the hip joint is the fulcrum, and the contraction of the adductor muscle is the effort.

Most of the limbs of the human body are articulated by third class lever. Each of the movements of the muscles for the various parts of the body are described by the following terms:

- Abductor: Moves a limb away from the midline.
- Adductor: Moves a limb toward the midline.
- Extensor: Increases the angle at a joint (extends a limb).
- Flexor: Decreases the angle at a joint (flexes a limb).

- Pronator: Turns a limb to face downwards.
- Supinator: Turns a limb to face upwards.
- Rotator: Rotates a limb.
- Sphincter: Closes an orifice or opening.

Heat Production

Heat is produced by the contractions of muscles. As much as 70% of body heat is produced by the metabolism of energy in muscle tissues. During exercise, blood is an essential element in the control of body temperature. When the body is overheating during physical exercise, blood takes the heat from the working muscles and redirects it to the skin. In contrary, when the internal heat of the body reaches too low a level, thermoreceptors in the skin relay a message to the hypothalamus in the brain. In response to this signal, the skeletal muscles contract and relax in an involuntary manner (shivering) increasing muscle activity to generate heat. Muscles are responsive to the external environmental conditions. Cold air increases muscle tone. Hot conditions have a relaxing effect on muscles.

Maintenance of Posture

Apart from enabling movement, muscles also maintain posture and body position. Sensory receptors in the muscles monitor the tension and length of the muscles and provide the nervous system with crucial information about the position of the body parts, therefore, enabling posture to be maintained. Muscles are never completely at rest, nor do they actually have to shorten in length, when they contract. The tension or tone produced as a result of these contractions between various opposing groups of muscle helps us to remain in a static position, even when we are asleep.

GENERAL FEATURES OF SKELETAL MUSCLE

Almost in every case, the skeletal muscles are attached to a bone with the help of tendons. A tendon is composed of densely packed nonelastic white fibrous connective tissue. At joints, the fibers of the tendon are affixed to the sarcolemma of the muscle fibers. To strengthen the junction, it is again surrounded by areolar tissue.

A single muscle fiber is a thread-like structure varying 1 to 3 inches in length. Microscopic examination reveals that the fiber consists of many myofibrils embedded in sarcoplasm and that is held together by a delicate membrane known as sarcolemma.

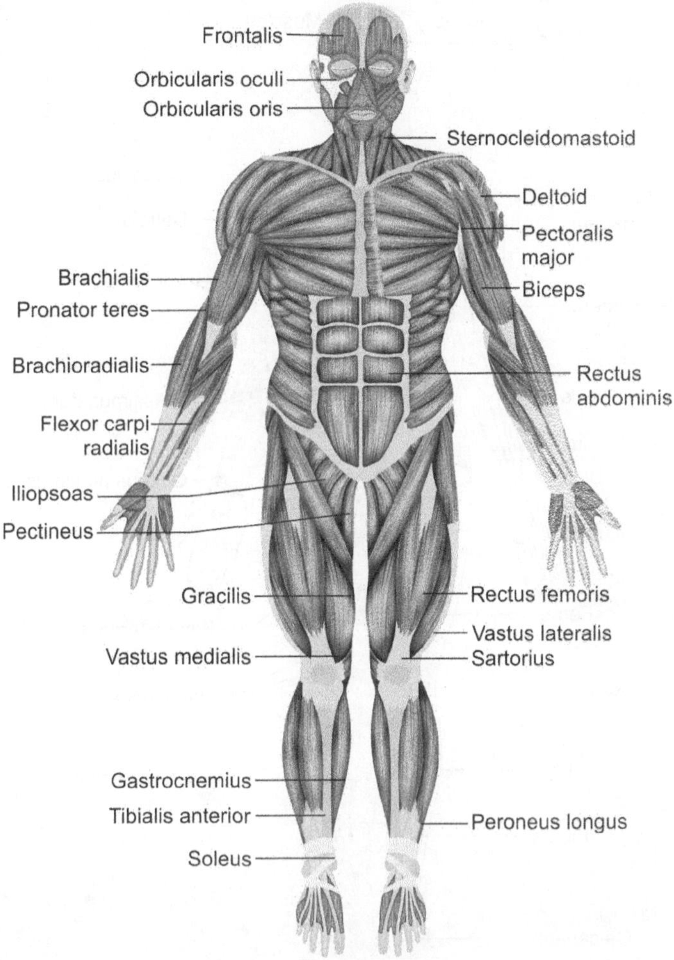

Fig. 3.1: Muscles of anterior view

Each fiber is enclosed within a thin connective tissue sheath called endomysium. The muscle fibers are bound into bundles within bundles. Each individual bundle of muscle fiber is enclosed in a fibrous tissue sheath called perimysium. The group of bundles that constitutes a complete muscle is in turn encased within a tougher connective tissue sheath called endomysium. A blood capillary is seen near each muscle fiber along with the endomysium. Anterior and posterior views of muscles are shown in Figures 3.1 and 3.2.

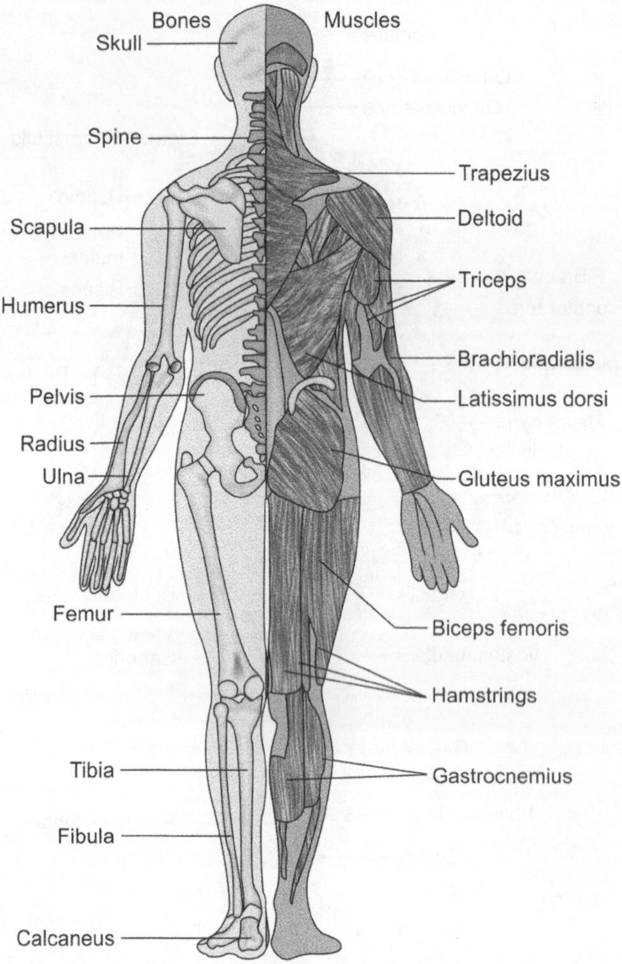

Fig. 3.2: Muscles of posterior view

HISTOLOGICAL STRUCTURE

The skeletal muscle fibers are cylindrical in shape. These elongated cells have multiple nuclei. In the bulk, the extent of the muscle fibers may be from:

- One end to the other
- One end to somewhere at midway
- Both the ends within the muscle having no attachments with either side.

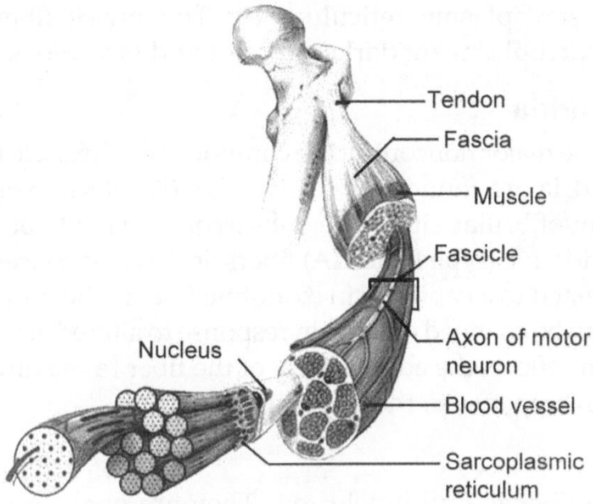

Fig. 3.3: Microscopic structure of muscle

Source: www.slideshare.net/LawrwnceJames/histo-muscle.

The length of the muscle fibers varies from 1.0 to 40 mm. The breadth varies from 0.01 to 0.1 mm. Albeit, the fiber size varies within the same muscle, yet there is some association between the thickness and size of the fibers and the amount of work to be done by the muscle. The thickness of the muscle fibers depends greatly on the nourishment of the individual. With the help of the regular exercise, total fiber volume increases along with the improvement of blood supply. The fiber number remains constant.

Sarcolemma

The transparent cell membrane of the muscle fiber is called as sarcolemma. With the help of electron micrography, it is observed that it is made up of plasmalemma and an extrinsic coat of amorphous material (similar to basement membrane). This amorphous layer is pierced and encircled by reticular fibers. The plasmalemma consists of two protein layers enclosing a lipid one having a thickness of 100A. Inside the plasmalemma, elongated multiple nuclei and transversely striated myofibrils are embedded in the sarcoplasm.

Sarcoplasm

The sarcoplasm contains numerous mitochondria, a small Golgi apparatus near each nucleus, myoglobin (protein pigment), lipid, glycogen, sarcoplasmic reticulum, etc. The muscle fibers that are richer in sarcoplasm are darker in color and vice versa.

Mitochondria

They are the major noncontractile components of muscle fibers. The mitochondria are found in two sites, i.e. (i) subsarcolemmal and (ii) intermyofibrillar sites. The subsarcolemmal site accumulates within oxidative (type I and IIA) fibers and a high concentration is often adjusted to a capillary in oxidative fibers. The mitochondrial volume can be changed quickly in response to altered activity levels. This again reflects the adaptability of the fiber to maximize its use of space in response to the physical activity.

Nuclei

A muscle fiber is multinucleated. They are oval- or elongated-shaped and situated just beneath sarcolemma. Because of its multinucleated condition, the muscle fiber is divided into a mosaic of overlapping regions or domains, each controlled by a nucleus. Within the domain, the nucleus controls the structural proteins. During postnatal development, muscle growth is rapid. More nuclei must be added to accommodate the increased fiber size at that time. When the incorporation of additional nuclei is inhibited, growth stunts (Rosenblatt et al. 1994). When nuclear distribution is measured, slow twitch (type I) fibers generally contain more nuclei than the fast twitch (type II) fibers. However, the volume per nucleus is higher in fast type than slow type fibers.

Myofibrils

These are the fine parallel filaments presents in sarcoplasm of the muscle fibers. The myofibrils extent through the entire length of the muscle fiber. Depending upon the length of the muscle fiber, the length of a myofibril varies from 1 to 4 cm with the diameter ranges from 0.2 to 2 microns. Studying the cross-section of a muscle fiber, it is found that the myofibrils are separated from one another by the sarcoplasm. Sometimes, some of the myofibrils are arranged in groups. These groups of myofibrils are known as Cohnheim's areas or fields.

Under the light microscope, it is found that myofibrils have alternate light and dark shades (transverse striations) and thick longitudinal strands. Electron micrography reveals that the longitudinal striation is due to the presence of the myofibrils of different thickness and transverse striation for the presence of alternate light and dark segments of longitudinally arranged elements.

Under polarized microscope, the dark band is anisotropic, hence the name A-band (sometimes called Q-band). The light band is isotropic hence the name I band (sometimes called J-band). This I-band is bisected at the midpoint by a thin darkly-stained line called as Z-line (sometimes called Dobie's line). It is also called as Krause's membrane. The portion of myofibril in between two Z-lines (in German, Zwischenscheibe = between disk) is called sarcomere. In certain exceptional preparations, central portion of the A- band is paler in color, called H-band (Hensen's line). At the midpoint of the H-band, there is a narrow dark line – the M-line or M-band. Myosin filaments are thickened here. At the peripheral dark portion of A-band where the myosin and actin filaments are overlapped, the portion is called O-band. A comparatively darker, thin, transverse line, called N-line, is found somewhere in the mid region of the I-band on the both the sides of the Z-line.

CHANGES DURING MUSCULAR CONTRACTION

After getting adequate stimulation the contraction of muscle starts. During the muscle contraction, the following changes occur:

- Electrical changes
- Physical changes
- Molecular changes
- Chemical changes
- Thermal changes.

Electrical Changes During Muscular Contraction

First of all, the muscle is stimulated and then electrical changes occur before the onset of the mechanical changes.

Resting Membrane Potential

Under resting condition, the potential difference between inside and outside of the cell is called as resting membrane potential. Through a suitable amplifier, if two electrodes of a cathode ray oscilloscope are placed on the surface of the muscle fiber, the potential difference will be zero. But if one of the electrodes is inserted inside the muscle fiber, a negative potential difference is noted. This potential difference is called as resting membrane potential and is constant. In our skeletal muscles, it is recorded as – 90mV.

Action Potential

When the muscle is stimulated an array of changes occurs in the membrane potential. It is called action potential. It occurs in two phases, viz. (i) depolarization and (ii) repolarization.

Depolarization

The moment when the impulse reaches the muscles, the resting membrane potential is altered. The inside of the muscle becomes positive and the outside becomes negative. The situation is called depolarization.

Repolarization

Within a short period of time, the muscle reestablishes the resting membrane potential, being interior of the muscle negatively and outside positively charged. This condition is called repolarization.

Physical Changes During Muscular Contraction

During muscular contraction, the muscle fiber shortens in length, increases in thickness, but the total volume remains same (or slightly increased). Muscular contraction may be of two types:

1. Isometric—when the length of the muscle fiber remains constant but the tension increases, it is called is isometric contraction.
2. Isotonic—when the muscle becomes shorter and thicker, it is called isotonic contraction.

Molecular Changes During Muscular Contraction

Excitation contraction coupling: Through a motor neuron, when the impulse reaches the neuromuscular junction, acetylcholine is released. Acetylcholine is responsible for the opening of ligand gated sodium channels. Thus, sodium ions enter the neuromuscular junction, leading to the development of end plate for the generation of action potential which spreads over sarcolemma through T tubules. The calcium ions move towards the actin filaments from sarcolemma to generate the contraction.

Sliding Theory

During muscular contraction the actin filaments slide over the myosin filaments forming the actomyosin complex.

From myosin filaments, each cross bridge has got three components, viz. (i) a hinge, (ii) an arm, and (iii) a head. After binding with active site of F-actin, the head of the myosin is tilted towards the arm and the actin filament is dragged along with it. This process is called power stroke. After tilting, the head immediately breaks away and combines with a new active site on the actin molecule. The tilting movement repeats again. The head of the cross-bridge bends back and forth and pulls the actin filaments towards the center of the sarcomere. In this process, all the actin filaments of both ends of sarcomere are pulled. Thus, the actin filaments of opposite sides overlap and form actomyosin complex.

Chemical Changes During Muscular Contraction

Breakdown of ATP

- The first step in the liberation of energy for muscular contraction is the breakdown of glycogen in the muscle fiber.
- The glycogen reacts with inorganic phosphate (Pi) and with the help of phosphorylase, splits up into glucose-1-phosphate.
- The process of uptake of the phosphate and its cleavage into glucose phosphate is called phosphorolysis.
- Glucose-1-phosphate is converted into glucose-6-phosphate. Glucose-6-phosphate is converted into fructose-6-phosphate, then into fructose-1-6-disphosphate and into two triose phosphates. The triose phosphate is finally converted into pyruvic acid.
- Pyruvic acid is reduced to lactic acid by reducing nicotinamide adenine dinucleotide (NAD.2H) and lactic dehydrogenase (in the absence of oxygen).
- Under anaerobic condition, one-fifth of the lactic acid is oxidized to CO_2 and H_2O; four-fifth are resynthesized into glycogen in liver.
- In the presence of oxygen, pyruvic acid is oxidized through Krebs tricarboxylic acid (TCA) cycle.
- In this cycle, one molecule of pyruvic acid loses one molecule of CO_2 and is converted into active acetyl coenzyme-A (acetate).
- The active acetate is metabolized through a series of reactions called citric acid cycle.
- Each molecule of pyruvic acid at each turn of the cycle, liberates three molecules of CO_2 and two molecules of H_2O.
- There is net production of 39 ATP per one hexose unit of glycogen metabolized. But 38 ATP are produced per oxidation

of one molecule of glucose metabolized. In anaerobic condition, 3 ATP are produced per hexose unit of glycogen metabolized and 2 ATP per molecule of glucose metabolized.

Thus, energy for muscular contraction is provided as ATP through:

- Anaerobic glycolysis leading to breakdown of glycogen and glucose to pyruvic acid and lactate.
- Oxidation of lactate to pyruvic acid and further oxidation of pyruvic acid in TCA cycle.
- Fatty acid oxidation through beta-oxidation.
- Creatine phosphate maintains the ATP level of the muscle.

Thermal Changes During Muscular Contraction

During muscular contraction, heat is produced in the muscle. The heat is released in different stages:

- **Resting heat:** In resting condition, the heat is produced in the muscle due to basal metabolic process. It is called resting heat.
- **Initial heat:** During muscular activity heat is produced in the following stages:
  - **Heat of activation:** Before the actual shortening of the muscle fibers, during the release of calcium ions from the L-tubules the heat is produced in the muscle fibers. It is called heat of activation.
  - **Heat of shortening:** During the contraction of muscle, the heat is produced due to the movement of cross bridges and breakdown of glycogen. It is called heat of shortening.
  - **Heat of relaxation:** During relaxation of muscle, the heat is released. It is called heat of relaxation.
- **Recovery heat:** After the end of muscular activities, some amount of heat is produced due to resynthesis of chemical substances. The heat is called recovery heat.

MUSCLE FIBER TYPES

Depending upon the contractile and metabolic characteristics, skeletal muscles have been divided into two groups:

1. Fast twitch fibers
2. Slow twitch fibers.

Fast Twitch Fibers

The fast twitch muscle fibers have the following characteristics:

- High capability for electrochemical transmission of action potentials.
- High myosin ATPase activity.
- Rapid Ca^{++} release and uptake by an efficient sarcoplasmic reticulum.
- High rate of cross bridge turnover.

All the above mentioned characteristics of the fast twitch fibers are responsible for the rapid generation of energy required for quick and powerful muscle actions. Their intrinsic speed of shortening and tension development ranges 3 to 5 times faster than slow twitch fibers. For energy transfer, the fast twitch muscle fibers follow a well-developed short-term glycolytic system. Sports events where forceful muscle actions are required like sprint, jumping events, throwing events, etc. fast twitch muscle fibers are beneficial with their anaerobic energy metabolism.

Slow Twitch Fibers

The slow twitch muscle fibers have the following characteristics:

- Relatively low myosin ATPase activity.
- Slower calcium handling ability and shortening speed.
- Glycolytic capacity less developed.
- Relatively larger and numerous mitochondria.

The slow twitch muscle fibers usually generate energy for ATP synthesis mainly through aerobic system of energy transfer. The red pigmentation of slow twitch fibers is due to large and numerous mitochondria combined with high levels of myoglobin. High concentration of mitochondrial enzymes is required to sustain aerobic metabolism. Slow twitch fibers are highly fatigue resistant and ideally suitable for prolonged aerobic exercise. In long and middle distance running, swimming and in other aerobic sports events slow twitch fibers provide adequate amount of energy keeping fatigue at bay for a long time.

MUSCLE STRENGTH AND POWER DIFFERENCES BETWEEN TWO SEXES

One of the most important male characteristics is the development of increasing musculature in puberty. Testosterone, a male sex hormone, is responsible for the muscular development in males, averaging about 50% increase in muscle mass over that in the females. This is associated with increased protein in other parts of the body as well. In young children up to 10 to 12 years old, boys are slightly stronger than girls. After these ages, during adolescence, biological and structural differences between boys and girls become marked and cultural influences encourage males to be physically active and girls to be docile. Subsequently the strength gap between the two sexes becomes wider. Generally, the differences of muscular strength and power between males and females continue to increase from the ages of 12 to 18 years. In fact, the males continue to improve the muscle strength and power with age, but females do not change significantly. By the time the average male reaches his college age, he gains almost twice the strength of the average females in the upper body and about one-third more in hips and legs.

AGE AND MUSCULAR STRENGTH

In determining muscular strength, physical growth and muscular activity play a major role. Force capacity of the muscle increases rapidly as a child grows physically from early age to adulthood. It is evident that the increase in muscle mass is positively correlated with force capacity. After reaching the physical maturation, application of overload training is essential to maintain the increment of muscle force. Otherwise, the muscles follow the general downward trend characteristic of other organ system with advancing age. Prolonged overload training enhances the muscular strength significantly during the early stages of adulthood. Maximum muscular strength is reached between the ages of 20 years in males and females and gradually declines about 20% of it at the age of 65 years.

BODY WEIGHT AND MUSCULAR STRENGTH

Persons with heavy body weight are reported to have more absolute strength and less relative strength than the persons with light body weight. When total strength is expressed per lb of body weight, the persons with lighter body weight have more strength per lb. It is found that gymnasts tend to be smaller in stature in comparison to footballers or shot putters. In gymnastics, a high level of strength is required per unit of body weight to best control and movement of the body weight. On the other hand, a large absolute level of strength is needed to footballers.

EFFECTS OF HEAVY RESISTANCE EXERCISE

Contractility is an important characteristic of skeletal muscle. When tension is generated in the contracting muscle, a large force is exerted on the pulling bones and connective tissues surrounding the skeletal joints. The tension is reflected in the structural make up of bones, ligaments, cartilage and tendons. As a result of work and exercise, structural changes occur in all these tissues. These adaptations to work and exercise are related to the changes in the functions of skeletal muscle.

An increase in protein synthesis results the increment of muscle fibers in length. Protein synthesis has an effect on the multiplication of myofibrils within the muscle fibers. Most of the researchers are of opinion that muscle hypertrophy is attributed to the increase of myofibrils rather than to the increase in muscle fibers. Nonetheless, some reports are also available which suggest that the number of fibers also increases. With the effects of the exercise, the stimulus for growth is repeated and continuous.

Muscle hypertrophy may also occur from the stimulus generated with the muscle stretching. Atrophy occurs at a relatively slower rate in the stretched muscle than in a muscle cast in a shortened position.

The collagen fibers in the connective tissue that surrounds the muscle act as a structural framework. As we know that the forces created by the contracting muscle fibers are transmitted to the bone by the connective tissues and tendons, it is easily understandable how muscle hypertrophy is associated with an increase in the collagen.

EFFECTS OF ANDROGENS ON HYPERTROPHY

There are several male sex hormones that collectively are called as androgens. They have two types of effects on the body:

1. Androgenic
2. Anabolic.

Androgenic effects are the development of secondary male sex characteristics, i.e. enlargement of the external genitalia and accessory sex organs, growth of body hair and enlargement of the vocal cords, resulting in a deeper voice.

The anabolic effects are growth and increment of protein synthesis in muscle tissue, resulting the increase in muscle growth. Testosterone is the most important hormone of this group. It is secreted by the male testes and adrenal cortex. A very lesser amount of this hormone is secreted by the female's adrenal cortex and ovaries. The difference in muscle size between males and females is due to the presence of testosterone in males in larger amounts.

The muscle hypertrophy depends greatly on the nature of the external work performed by an individual. It is evident that the lifting heavy loads are associated with gains in muscle size. During heavy work, testosterone is secreted in greater amount. Sutton and Tonskins (1974) reported that after a heavy workout in water, the male swimmers showed the increment of testosterone levels as well as their muscle size. Fahey (1976) had the same opinion regarding college males after weight training. Although, both males and females respond to training in terms of strength and hypertrophy, males exceed females in proportional increase in muscle girth (Brown and Wilmore, 1974).

MUSCLE STRENGTH AND MOVEMENT VELOCITY

Quick movement of the body is the effect of increased muscle strength. Performances in different sports events are largely depended on the rapid movement of the body. With the help of strength training regularly, sports persons involve in increasing muscle strength. Nelson and Fahrney (1965), and Nelson and Jordan (1969) were of the opinion that when a maximum strength was based on an isometric contraction and was related to movement time (MT) of the limb, stronger individuals might move faster. Nevertheless, this is not always the case (Smith and Whitley, 1963). It was reported that when maximum strength was based on a concentric contraction in the bench press lift and a relationship was determined between strength and movement time with different loads from heavy to light, significant association was found. In fact, stronger individuals might move almost twice the loads of weaker individuals and at the same velocity.

In sports performances also, quick movement and power, especially with heavy loads involving either body weight and/or external weight, require a high level of muscle strength. The larger the load to be moved in athletes, the greater the advantage of being strong.

STRENGTH AND POWER RELATIONSHIP IN PERFORMANCE

Power is the physical component involved when an explosive movement occurs. It is the amount of work performed in a unit of time. Work can be defined as the application of force through a distance. The formula for work is:

$$W = F \times D$$

Where, W is work done, F is force (a constant force); D is distance (through which the force is moved). Accordingly to CGS system, the absolute unit of work is erg and in FPS system it is ftlb. In CGS system, the practical unit of work is Joule and in FPS system, it is ftlb.

As mentioned earlier, power is the work done in a unit of time. So the formula is:

$$\text{Power} = \frac{\text{Work}}{\text{Time}} = \frac{F \times D}{t}$$

In explosive sports, force possesses a factor of acceleration or change in velocity ($F = M \times A$; where, M = mass, A = acceleration). The power may be formulated as:

$$\text{Power} = \frac{M \times A \times D}{t}$$

Force generated by muscular contraction provides the acceleration given to the mass (M) or body weight in running events or jumping. Increasing force and speed, acceleration required to complete the work will increase, but the time will be decreased. When acceleration is increased and time is decreased, power increases.

Athletes must have adequate power to perform in sports events. In football, linemen are tall and large, as their large size provides them a greater capacity for power, which is essential for overcoming the opponents or blocking. On the other hand, in 100 m sprints, the total amount of power generated by a moving body is not so important, as the time required moving a specific distance is the prime. The same is the case of fencing too. In these events, power relative to body weight is more important. In such events, where running speed and quickness are essential, large muscle mass may be detrimental. Nonetheless, with the help of overloading training, the increasing muscle size may increase the force as well as acceleration.

A sprinter should reduce his/her body weight as he/she requires maximum acceleration and movement speed. A defender in football should increase muscle mass adequately to get maximum absolute power. In case of linemen in the same ball game, some absolute power may be sacrificed to get quickness or acceleration. In fact, the combination of both absolute power and acceleration is desirable for best performance in this event. Defensive backers desire more relative power than the absolute power. In these positions the players must move quickly. An offensive backer must have both absolute power to overcome a tackler and relative power to avoid the chase of intended tacklers.

CHAPTER 4

Effects of Exercise on Cardiovascular System

CARDIOVASCULAR SYSTEM

Cardiovascular system includes the heart and the blood vessels. The heart pumps the blood into the blood vessels which circulate the blood throughout our body. Blood transports oxygen from the lungs to the tissue and carbon dioxide from the tissue to the lungs and nutrients from the elementary tract to the tissues and cell waste materials to the kidneys.

The Heart

It is roughly a cone-shaped hollow muscular organ of about 10 cm long, weighing about 225 g in women and 310 g in men and is about the size of our closed fist. The heart is in the thoracic cavity in the mediastinum between the lungs. It lies obliquely, slightly more to the left side than the right, base is above and apex below (Fig. 4.1). The organs associated with the heart are as follows:

- Superiorly: The great blood vessels, i.e. the aorta, superior vena cava, pulmonary artery and pulmonary veins.
- Inferiorly: The apex lies on the central tendon of the diaphragm.
- Posteriorly: The esophagus, trachea, left and right bronchus, descending aorta, inferior vena cava and thoracic vertebrae.
- Laterally: The lungs.
- Anteriorly: The sternum, ribs and intercostal muscles.

Interior Structure

The heart is divided into a right and left side by the septum, a partition consisting of myocardium covered by endocardium. Each side is divided by an atrioventricular valve into an upper chamber the atrium, and a lower chamber, the ventricle. The right atrioventricular valve has three flaps (tricuspid) and the left atrioventricular valve (mitral/bicuspid valve) has two flaps.

Papillary muscles are also present in the heart. Papillary muscles are responsible for opening of the valves and are five in numbers. Chordae tendineae are the tendons of the papillary muscles. They prevent the valves from opening upwards into the atria.

Cardiac muscle: The myocardium is composed of a specialized cardiac muscle tissue found only in heart. Myocardium is thickest at the apex and thins out towards the base. Branching cells and intercalated disks are the characteristics of the cardiac muscle.

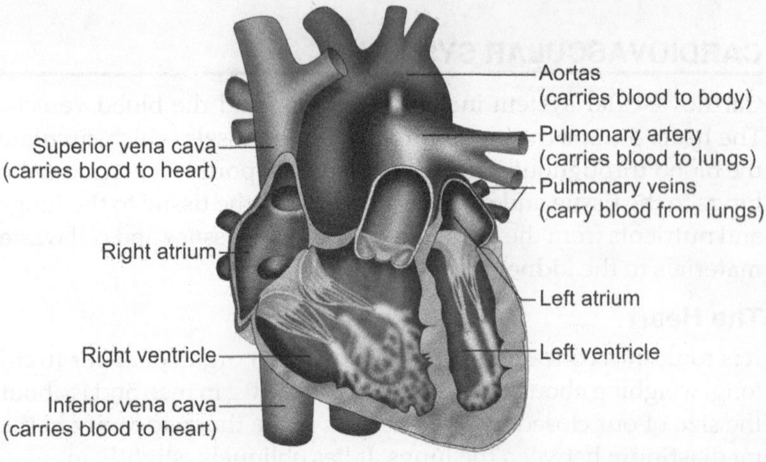

Fig. 4.1: Structure of the heart

Heart Sounds

During the action of the heart, two sounds are heard. The first sound occurs due to the closing of atrioventricular valve and contraction of the ventricles. It is long and dull like 'lubb'. The second sound occurs due to closure of aortic and pulmonary valves. It is short and sharp and sounds like 'dupp'.

EFFECT OF EXERCISE ON CARDIOVASCULAR SYSTEM

Due to the effect of exercise, some changes occur in the cardiovascular system of our body. Various effects of exercise on cardiovascular system are given as follows:

Effect on Blood

During exercise, a mild hypoxia is developed which stimulates the juxtaglomerular apparatus to secrete erythropoietin. This stimulates the bone marrow causing the release of red blood cells. During exercise, the increased carbon dioxide content in blood decreases the pH of blood.

Effect on Blood Volume

During exercise, more heat is produced, activating the thermoregulatory system of our body. It causes secretion of large amount of sweat leading to:

- Reduction of blood volume
- Fluid loss
- Hemoconcentration
- Dehydration due to severe exercise.

Size of Heart

During exercise, excessive workload is imposed upon the heart. With prolonged and systemic exercises, the heart becomes enlarge to cope with the excessive workload. This hypertrophy of the heart in athletes is caused by physiological processes. In fact, the mass and volume of the heart gradually increase with long-term aerobic training. Greater left ventricular end-diastolic volume is also noted along with increase in the size of the left ventricular cavity (eccentric hypertrophy) and modest thickening of its walls (concentric hypertrophy). This hypertrophied athletic heart is more efficient with greater increase in stroke volume. Stroke volume is the amount of blood pumped by each ventricle during each beat, normal volume is 70 mL. This hypertrophied athletic heart should not be misunderstood with the cardiac enlargement of patients with hypertension. In hypertension, the heart chronically works against an excessive resistance to blood flow. This stretches the heart muscle, which generates compensatory force to overcome the added resistance to systolic ejection. In addition to ventricular dilation, individual muscle cells hypertrophied to adjust to the increased myocardial work imposed by the hypertensive state. In untreated hypertension, myocardial fibers stretch beyond their optimal length and the dilated heart weakens which eventually fails. To the pathologists, this (hypertrophied) heart represents an enlarged distended and functionally inadequate organ unable to deliver enough blood to satisfy minimal resting requirements.

Research Findings

Research has compared male competitive swimmers, long distance runners, wrestlers and shot putters during their competitive seasons with untrained college men. The swimmers and runners represented athletes participating in isotonic or endurance events; the wrestlers and short putters represented isometric or resistance-trained, power athletes. Heart structure differs among athletes related to the nature of exercise training. For instance, in the swimmers, left ventricular volume averaged 181 mL and mass equalled 308 g; the nonathletic controls averaged 101 mL for ventricular volume and 211g for ventricular mass. The resistance trained athletes had thickened ventricular walls, while those of endurance athletes remained within the normal range.

Possible Explanation of Hypertrophied Heart in Athletes

Myocardial structural and dimensional adaptations to regular exercise generally reflect specific training demands. Within a day or two of the onset of endurance training, the plasma volume increases. This increased plasma volume probably produces intraventricular enlargement or eccentric hypertrophy. Increased plasma volume, coupled with a decreased heart rate and increased myocardial complainer, dilates the left ventricular cavity. In contrast, male and female resistance trained athletes possess the largest intraventricular septum, ventricular wall thickness and ventricular mass, with little enlargement in the left ventricle's internal cavity. These athletes do not experience volume overload with training. Instead, they encounter acute episodes of significantly elevated arterial blood pressure from high forces generated by a limited mass of skeletal muscle. An increase in ventricular wall thickness (which generally falls within the normal range when expressed as ventricular mass per unit body size, particularly fat-free body mass) compensates for the additional after load on the left ventricle without affecting ventricular cavity size.

The **athlete's heart** does not represent a dysfunctional organ. Rather, it demonstrates normal systolic and diastolic functions and superior functional capacity for stroke volume and cardiac output.

- Impulses from proprioceptors are present in the exercising muscles. These impulses act through higher centers and increase the heart rate.
- Increased carbon dioxide tension: It acts through medullary centers.

- Rise in body temperature: It acts on cardiac centers through hypothalamus. Increased body temperature stimulates SA node directly.
- The circulating catecholamines, which are secreted in large quantities during exercise.

Effect on Plasma Volume

A 12 to 20% increase in plasma volume, in the absence of changes in red blood cell mass, occurs after 3 to 6 aerobic training sessions. In fact, a significant change takes place within 24 hours of the first exercise bout, with expansion of the extracellular fluid volume requiring several weeks. Intravascular volume expansion directly relates to increased synthesis and retention of plasma albumin. A plasma volume increase enhances circulating reserve and contributes to increased end-diastolic volume, stroke volume, oxygen transport and temperature regulation during exercise. The expanded plasma volume returns to pertaining levels within 1 week after training ceases.

Effect on Stroke Volume

The effect of exercise on stroke volume is highly dependent on hydrostatic pressure effects. At rest, in erect position, stroke volume in healthy adults generally varies between 60 to 100 mL/beat, while maximum stroke volume approximates 100 to 120 mL/beat. During exercising in erect position stroke volume increases curvilinearly (Mountain et al. 1997) and early with the workload until it reaches a mean maximum value increasingly only slightly thereafter. During exercise, there is an increase in stroke volume resulting from both the Frank-Starling mechanism and a decreased end-systolic volume. In moderate exercise, the heart rate increases upto 180 beats/min. It reaches 240 to 260 beats/min in severe muscular exercise.

Effect on Heart Rate

In human, the normal heart rate is 72 beats per minute. It generally increases immediately following exercise. It is noticed that heart rate is increased slightly even before the onset of exercise. Presumably this is due to the influence of the cerebral cortex on the medullary cardiac centers which reduces vagal tone. At the first minute of exercise, a short rise of heart rate is recorded. But after that, the rate of rise is slightly decreased. The maximum rise is achieved within 4 to 5 minutes of exercise. There is a linear relationship between heart rate and workload or power output. If the exercise is further continued, a plateau is observed, though workload and time vary person-to-person. The rate of rise of heart rate is slower in trained athletes. In moderate exercise, the heart rate increases upto 180 beats/min. It reaches 240 to 260 beats/min in severe muscular exercise. The maximum heart rate attained during exercise depends upon the following factors:

- Emotion
- Environmental temperature
- Humidity
- Physical conditions of the individual.

Explanation for the Increase in Heart Rate

It is claimed that nervous and chemical factors are responsible for the increase in heart rate. Anticipatory heart rate or just before exercise, initial rise of heart rate is due to the influence of cerebral cortex and other higher brain centers. With the onset of exercise, the increase of heart rate may be due to:

- Reflexes originating in the receptors of moving joints or contracting muscles.
- Stimulation of chemoreceptors in muscles by the acid metabolites.
- Sympatheticoadrenal activation causing secretion of much larger amount of epinephrine in blood.
- Rise of blood temperature.
- Stimulation of stretch receptors in atrium by the rapid venous return in heart, thus causing brain bridge – reflex.

The return of heart rate to initial resting level depends on:

- The intensity of workload
- Physical condition of the individual.

After the cessation of exercise, the rapidity of return of heart rate is considered as a test for physical fitness. The recovery period is very short for trained athletes or physically fit persons, whereas, for sedentary people this recovery period is rather prolonged.

Effect on Cardiac Output

Cardiac output is directly proportional to heart rate. During exercise, the cardiac output is increased. It is reported that in case of trained athletes, the maximum cardiac output is 30 L/min, with oxygen uptake of 4 L/min. The non-athletes have the average cardiac output of 22 L/min with oxygen uptake of 33 L/min. During exercise, the cardiac output is the result of the increase in stroke volume and heart rate. Increased heart rate is because of vagal withdrawal and the increased stroke volume is due to increased force of contraction. Though modern literature claims that the diastolic size of the heart is decreased during exercise so that the increased stroke volume cannot be caused by greater stretching. Researchers claimed that the increased cardiac output during exercise was mostly due to increase of heart rate.

Effect of Venous Return

During exercise, venous return is remarkably increased. The reasons may be due to:

- Milking or massaging action of skeletal muscles: The alternate contraction and relaxation of the skeletal muscles during exercise acts as a booster pump for flowing of blood towards the heart. Valves are there in the vein. During contraction, blood is squeezed out from the vein towards the heart through the valves. During relaxation of the muscles, it allows to fill blood. Albeit, this pumping mechanism depends upon the intensity and type of exercise.
- Respiratory movements: Respiratory movements exert a sucking effect on the right heart and great veins causing greater venous return. During inspiration, the thoracic cavity becomes enlarge causing the fall of interthoracic pressure. Rapid return of blood into the heart is caused by this fall of intrathoracic pressure on one hand and the increase of pressure on the anterior abdominal wall on the other hand. Expiration has got the opposite effect.
- Contraction of limb veins: During exercise, the limb veins undergo splanchnic vasoconstriction, facilitating rapid venous return to the heart.

Effect on Blood Pressure

During moderate isotonic exercise, the systolic blood pressure is increased due to increased heart rate and stroke volume. The diastolic pressure is not altered much as the peripheral resistance is not altered much during moderate isotonic exercise. In severe exercise, the systolic blood pressure increases enormously, but the diastolic pressure decreases. The fall in diastolic blood pressure in isotonic muscular contraction is due to the reduction of vasodilatation caused by metabolites further reducing the peripheral resistance. On the other hand, the rise of arterial blood pressure during severe muscular exercise is due to:

- Increase in cardiac output causing greater distention of aorta and large arteries.
- Increase in heart rate.
- Compensatory vasoconstriction in the nonactive organs and vasodilatation in the active organs.

It is rather difficult to generalize the nature of blood pressure rise as the changes of blood pressure mostly depend on the following factors:

- Type of activity
- Speed of the activity
- Duration of the activity
- Physical condition of the individual.

Blood Pressure After Exercise

During exercise, large quantities of metabolic end products are produced. These metabolic end products accumulate in the tissues, especially in the skeletal muscles. These substances cause vasodilatation. So after exercise, the blood pressure falls slightly below the resting level. Nonetheless, the pressure returns to the resting level quickly as soon as the metabolic end products are removed from the muscles.

Effect on Blood Flow to Skeletal Muscles

During exercise, the blood flow to skeletal muscles increases greatly. In resting condition, the blood supply to the skeletal muscles is 3 to 4 mL per 100 g of the muscle per minute. This increases upto 60 to 80 mL in moderate exercise and upto 90 to 120 mL in severe exercise. The circulation during exercise is adjusted in such a way that the active muscles and vital organs get greater proportion of blood supply than the inactive and nonvital organs. In fact, active muscles get more blood supply during exercise, due to decrease of vascular resistance caused by accumulation of metabolic end products. During exercise, increased accumulation of carbon dioxide, lactic acid, adenosine, intracellular K^+ and histamine causes sudden lack of oxygen.

During exercise, blood flow may stop temporarily, when the muscles contract. This may be due to compression of blood vessels during contraction but the blood flow increases in between the contractions.

It is important that sometimes the blood supply to muscles increases even during the preparation for exercise. This may be due to vasodilatation in muscles caused by sympathetic nerve activity.

Certain factors are responsible for the increase of blood supply to muscles during exercise by means of vasodilatation. These are:

- Excess of carbon dioxide
- Hypoxia
- Metabolic end products like lactic acid
- Potassium ions
- Rise in temperature
- Adrenaline secreted from adrenal medulla
- Increased sympathetic cholinergic activity.

EXERCISE STRENGTH TESTING FOR DIAGNOSIS OF CORONARY HEART DISEASES

Coronary heart disease continues to be the leading cause of death worldwide. Of those persons who die suddenly of coronary heart disease, 50% of men and 64% of women have had no previous signs or symptoms. Accurate assessment and risk stratification of patients with coronary heart disease are crucial in identifying patients at greatest risk for coronary events. Thus, clinicians must be knowledgeable about the many forms of cardiac diagnostic testing available. The coronary angiography is invasive and expensive, and involves a risk for acute myocardial infarction, stroke, arrhythmias. This imaging method is not considered a first-line diagnostic study in patients at low risk for heart disease.

Stress Test

- Stress testing is one of the most commonly used methods of non-invasive assessment of coronary artery disease.
- Stress testing involves the use of exercise (for patients who are physically able) or drugs such as vasodilators and dobutamine (for patients who are physically unable to exercise) to increase myocardial demand and is used to determine the presence of ischemia.
- Assessment data are collected by using continuous ECG monitoring, echocardiography, nuclear imaging, or various combinations of these 3 methods.

Exercise Stress Testing

- Strenuous exercise increases heart rate, stroke volume, and cardiac output, and activates the sympathetic nervous system, resulting in vasoconstriction of most vasculature except that of the exercising muscle and cerebral and coronary vessels.
- Release of norepinephrine and increased levels of renin result in increased cardiac contractility.
- During exercise, coronary blood flow increases.
- Obstructive coronary artery disease prohibits adequate coronary blood flow to the affected area of the myocardium and ischemia occurs.

Respiration During Exercise

- Dynamic exercise-ventilation increases linearly over the mild-to-moderate range, then increases rapidly in intense exercise.
- Workload at which rapid ventilation occures is called the ventilatory breakpoint (together with lactate threshold).

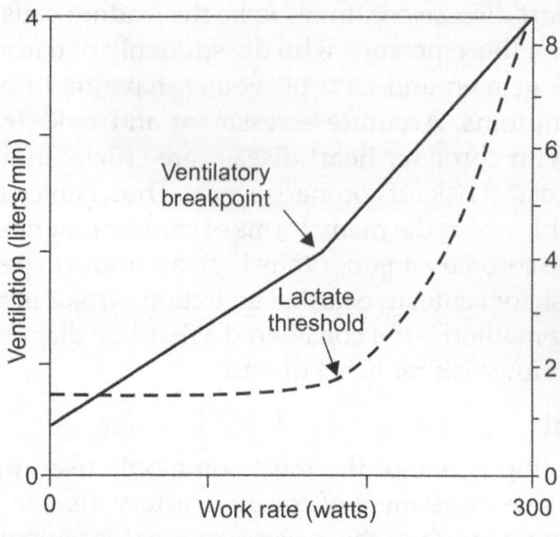

Fig. 4.2: Relationship of work rate and blood lactate concentration

Blood Pressure Rise in Exercise

- Systolic blood pressure increases upto 150 to 170 mm Hg during dynamic exercise; diastolic pressure rarely alters.
- Isometric exercises—Systolic blood pressure may increase upto 250 mm Hg, and diastolic blood pressure can reach upto 180 mm Hg.

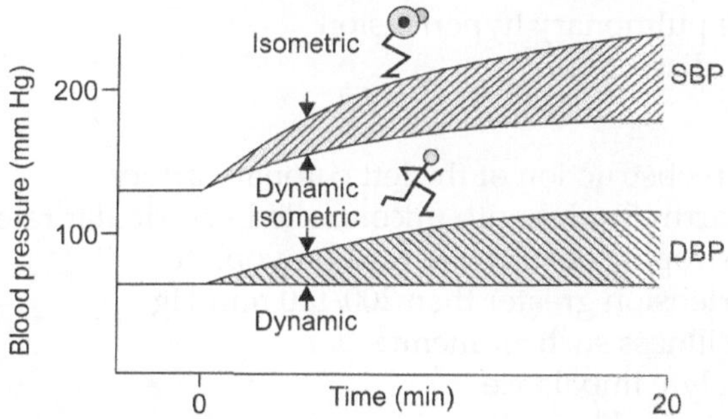

Fig. 4.3: Relationship of exercise and blood pressure

Postexercise Phase

- Vagal reactivation
  - Important cardiac deceleration mechanism.
- Increase in well-trained athletes.
- Blunted in cardiac failure.
- About 70 to 80% occlusion - detection by exercise strength testing.
- Sign of coronary artery disease can exist with a negative exercise stress test.
- Exercise stress testing is therefore a useful way to assess for evidence of myocardial ischemia and exercise capacity.
- Exercise stress testing often involves use of a treadmill or bicycle ergometer.
- In order to participate in an exercise stress test, patients must be alert and oriented and have adequate coordination.
- Advanced age, poor functional capacity, poor balance, joint or back pain, and generalized deconditioning are typically contraindications to treadmill testing; in these instances, pharmacological testing may be used.

Contraindications to Stress Testing

Absolute

- Congestive heart failure
- Uncontrolled cardiac arrhythmias
- Severe aortic stenosis
- Unstable angina
- Myocardial infarction within the past 2 days
- Acute pulmonary embolus
- Myocarditis

- Severe pulmonary hypertension
- Aortic dissection.

Relative

- Known obstruction of the left coronary artery
- Tachyarrhythmias with uncontrolled ventricular rate
- Hypertrophic obstructive cardiomyopathy
- Hypertension greater than 200/110 mm Hg
- Acute illness such as anemia
- Electrolyte imbalance
- Uncontrolled hyperthyroidism.

Indications (Flowchart 4.1)

- Patients with symptoms or prior history of CAD
  - Initial evaluation with suspected or known CAD
  - Known CAD with change in status (crescendo)
  - Low risk, unstable angina 8 to 12 hours after presentation free of symptoms (rule out time)
  - Intermediate risk, unstable angina, 2 to 3 days free of active ischemia.
- Post-MI
  - Prognostic assessment
  - Activity prescription
  - Evaluation of medical therapy
  - Before beginning cardiac rehabilitation.
- Before stress testing begins, advanced cardiac life support equipment should be on standby. Leads are placed on the patient for 12-lead ECG, and baseline values are obtained. Baseline vital signs are assessed along with the patient's history and list of medications.
- Medications such as digoxin, calcium channel blockers, and beta-blockers may produce ST-segment depression or prevent the patient from reaching the target heart rate. If safe to do so, administration of these medications should be stopped 24 to 48 hours before the stress test is done.

Indications For Terminating Exercise Testing

Absolute

- Acute myocardial infarction
- Moderate to severe angina
- Symptomatic decrease in systolic blood pressure despite an increase in workload

Flowchart 4.1: Indications of stress testing

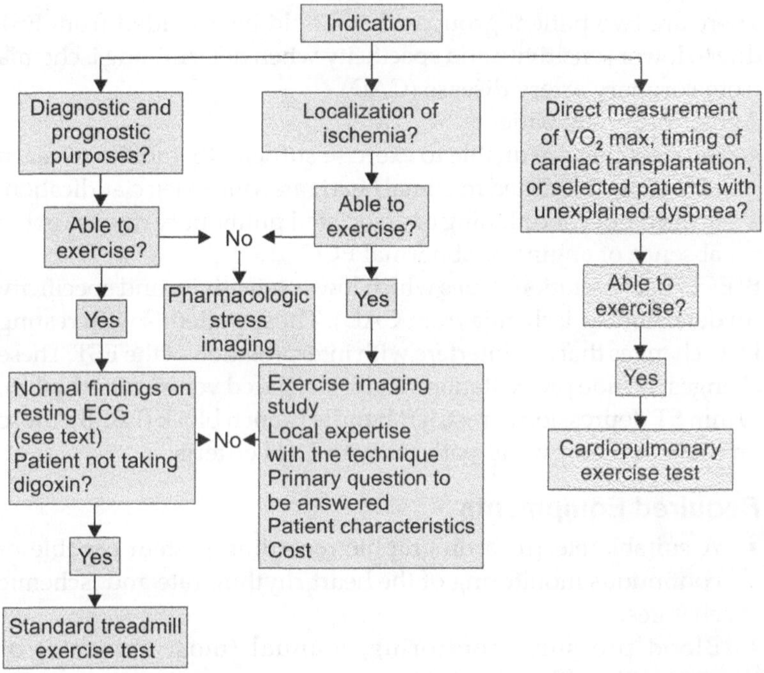

- Arrhythmias such as second- or third-degree atrioventricular block, ventricular tachycardia, frequent premature ventricular contractions, atrial fibrillation
- Signs of poor perfusion including pallor, cyanosis, or cold, clammy skin
- Severe dyspnea
- Ataxia, vertigo, visual or gait problems, or confusion
- Patient requests to stop.

Relative

- Decrease in systolic blood pressure greater than 10 mm Hg from baseline blood pressure, despite an increase in workload, in the absence of signs and symptoms
- Increasing angina
- Hypertensive response (systolic blood pressure >260 mm Hg, diastolic blood pressure >115 mm Hg)
- Fatigue, shortness of breath, wheezing, leg cramps, or claudication.

Exercise Stress Test Limitations

There are two patient groups who should be excluded from EST due to lower sensitivity and specificity when determining ischemia from coronary artery disease (CAD).

A: Inappropriate patients

- Patients that are unable to exercise sufficiently (ability to reach 85% of age predicted maximal heart rate) due to leg claudication, arthritis, deconditioning or associated pulmonary disease in the absence of angina or abnormal ECG.

B: ECG interpretation issues which lower sensitivity and specificity (in determining ischemia from CAD). Those patient's with resting ECG changes that can interfere with interpretation of the EST. These changes include preexcitation syndrome, paced ventricular rhythm, >1mm ST depression at rest, left bundle branch block (LBBB), those on digoxin therapy and patients with LVH criteria.

Required Equipments

- A suitable electrocardiographic recording system capable of continuous monitoring of the heart rhythm, rate and ischemic changes.
- Blood pressure monitoring, manual (most accurate) or automatic with a variety of cuff sizes.
- Electronic treadmill that ranges in speed between 1.6 km/hr and 12.8 km/hr and gradient range of 0 to 22%. Treadmills should have a front rail and at least one side rail for safety and should be fitted with an emergency stop button.
- Automated external defibrillator (tested daily) and other emergency equipment readily.

Test Procedure Skin Preparation and ECG Placement Available

- After a standard resting 12-lead recording, a modified limb lead ECG should be recorded. Compare the modified ECG to the standard ECG prior to exercise to assess for any significant ECG differences.
- Modifications should be made to the limb leads by moving them onto the torso. The left and right arm should be placed as close to the shoulder as possible while the leg electrodes should be placed below the umbilicus.

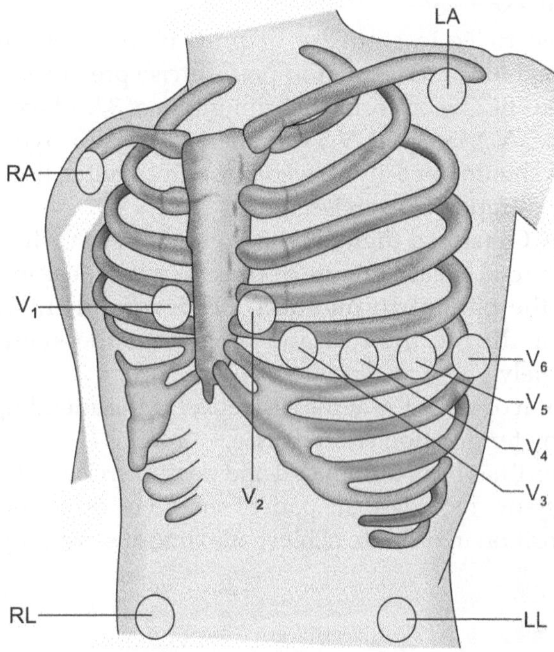

Fig. 4.4: Exercise stress testing and data collection

Performing the EST and Data Collection (Fig. 4.4)

- Explain the procedure fully, detailing what is going to happen during the exercise stress testing (EST).
- Inform the patient that in order to perform the EST, unrestricted access to the chest area will be required.
- Ensure a consent form has been read and signed once the procedure has been explained to the patient.
- The patient should be covered with a gown during the procedure to ensure their modesty.
- Once the patient has been set-up, record a standard resting supine12-lead ECG.
- Change the limb lead positions and record a modified limb lead resting supine 12-lead ECG.
- Demonstrate the correct use of the exercise equipment to the patient before commencing the test.
- Record the patient's blood pressure:
  - prior to starting exercise as a baseline reference
  - once during every stage of exercise

  - at peak exercise
  - at least twice in recovery or until blood pressure has returned to values similar to pre-exercise pressure.
- Continuous ECG monitoring of a minimum of 3 leads covering anterior (V_1, V_2), lateral (I, V_5) and inferior (II, aVF) myocardial territories should be easily viewed through a digital display for the entire duration of exercise.
- 12-lead ECGs (stored digitally, hard copy or both) should be taken at the end of each minute of exercise and at peak exercise.
- Instruct the patient to mention the development of any symptoms during the test and document the symptoms appropriately.
- Termination of an EST is at the discretion of the attending staff should any termination criteria arise.
- Once an EST has been terminated and peak exercise ECG's and blood pressure recorded, the patient should be positioned in a supine position in order to achieve maximum sensitivity.

CHAPTER 5

Effects of Exercise on Respiratory System

Respiration is the process by which oxygen is taken in and carbon dioxide is given out. Respiration occurs in two stages, viz. (i) inspiration and (ii) expiration.

Inspiration: It is a process by which atmospheric air enters into the lungs. During normal breathing, inspiration (inhalation) is an active process.

Expiration: It is a process by which air leaves from the lungs. Expiration (exhalation) is a passive process.

While passing through the lungs, the atmospheric air (inspired air) delivers oxygen to the blood in the pulmonary capillaries and takes away carbon dioxide from the body in exchange. Thus, blood provides the transport system for these gases between lungs and the cells of the body. Respiration is of two types, viz.

External respiration: Exchange of respiratory gases (oxygen and carbon dioxide) between alveoli of lungs and blood in pulmonary capillaries is called external respiration. The phases of external respiration include:

- Air entering the lungs
- Oxygen leaving the lungs and entering the pulmonary blood
- Blood transporting oxygen to all the cells of the body
- Blood transporting carbon dioxide to the lungs
- Carbon dioxide leaving the blood and entering the lungs
- Carbon dioxide leaving the lungs.

Internal respiration: The exchange of gases between blood and tissues is called internal respiration. It includes only the utilization of oxygen and the production of carbon dioxide and other metabolites by the cells.

EFFECTS OF EXERCISE ON RESPIRATORY SYSTEM

Muscular exercise brings about a lot of changes on respiratory system of the body (Fig. 5.1). The degree of changes depends on the severity and duration of exercise.

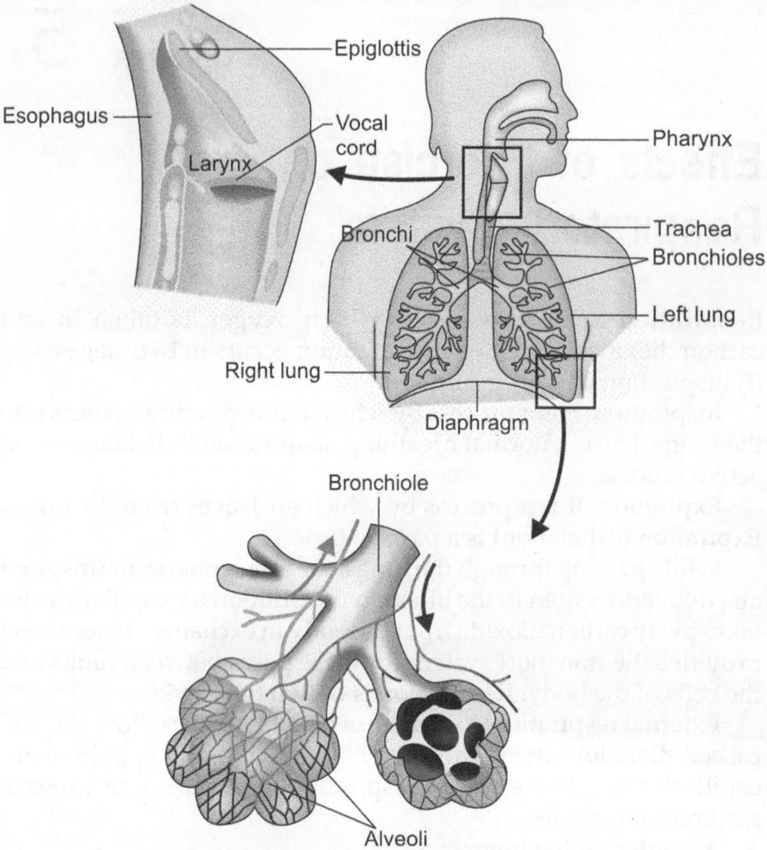

Fig. 5.1: Respiratory system

Pulmonary ventilation: It is the amount of air that enters and leaves the lungs in 1 minute. It is the product of tidal volume and respiratory rate. Tidal volume is the volume of air breathed in and out during each respiratory cycle. During exercise, it increases from a resting volume of 0.5 L to around 3 L. During exercise, respiratory rate increases from a resting rate of 12 to 20 breaths/min. At rest, the pulmonary ventilation value is around 5 to 8 L/min for normal healthy individual. In a short period of hard work, it may exceed 130 L/min for females and 180 L/min for males. In well-trained athletes, it may go over 200 L/min which is approximately more than 30 times the resting value. Pulmonary ventilation not only increases during exercise, but also has a linear relationship between this increase and the amount of oxygen absorbed, and the amount of carbon dioxide produced per minute.

The respiratory rate increases during moderate exercise to about 30 beats/min and tidal volume increases to about 2000 mL. Therefore, the pulmonary ventilation increases to about 60 L/min during moderate exercise. In severe muscular exercise, it rises till further upto 100 L/min.

Factors Affecting Pulmonary Ventilation

- **Higher centers:** During the onset of exercise, the rate, rhythm and depth of respiration increases. In some cases, anticipation of exercise increases even before exercise. This is obviously a psychic phenomenon due to the activation of higher center of brain. This is formed by groups of nerve cells. They are situated in the brainstem, in the medulla oblongata and the pons varolii. It is reported that the interrelationship between these groups of cells is complex during exercise. In the medulla, inspiratory neurons and expiratory neurons are situated. Neurons in the pneumotaxic and apneustic centers, situated in the pons, influence the inspiratory and expiratory neurons of the medulla. Motor impulses leaving the respiratory center pass in the phrenic and intercostal muscles respectively.
- **Chemoreceptors:** These are the receptors that respond to changes in the partial pressures of oxygen and carbon dioxide in the blood and cerebrospinal fluid. These receptors are the sensory nerve endings which are highly sensitive to chemical changes in blood. They are located centrally and peripherally.
- **Central hemoreceptors:** They are situated on the surface of the medulla oblongata and are bathed in cerebrospinal fluid. During exercise, when the arterial PCO_2 rises, the central chemoreceptors respond by stimulating the respiratory centers, increasing ventilation of the lungs and reducing the arterial PCO_2. The sensitivity of the central chemoreceptors to raised arterial PCO_2 is the most important factor in maintaining homeostasis of blood gases in health.
- **Peripheral chemoreceptors:** They are situated in the arch of the aorta and in the carotid bodies. They are more sensitive to small rises in arterial PCO_2 than to identically low arterial PO_2 levels. Nerve impulses, generated in the peripheral chemoreceptors,

are conveyed by the glossopharyngeal and vagus nerve to the medulla and stimulate the respiratory centers.

- **Proprioceptors:** During exercise, proprioceptors are activated and send impulses to cerebral cortex through the somatic afferent nerves. Cerebral cortex, in turn, causes hyperventilation by sending impulses to the medullary respiratory centers.
- **Body temperature:** During exercise, body temperature increases causing the increase in ventilation by stimulating the respiratory centers.
- **Acidosis:** In blood, a low pH results from a high hydrogen ion concentration is called acidosis. During exercise, when the by-products of cellular activity, such as carbon dioxide, lactic acid, phosphoric acid, etc. are being produced, the pH becomes more acidic, around 7.05. This acidosis stimulates the respiratory centers resulting in hyperventilation.

DIFFUSING CAPACITY FOR OXYGEN

The diffusing capacity is defined as the volume of gas that diffuses through the respiratory membrane each minute for a pressure gradient of 1 mm Hg. Pressure gradient is the difference between the partial pressure of a gas in the alveoli and the partial pressure of that gas in the blood in the pulmonary capillary. Diffusing capacity is directly proportional to the pressure gradient.

Diffusing capacity for oxygen is 21 mL/min/mm Hg in resting condition. It is noticed that the diffusing capacity for carbon dioxide is 20 times more than that of oxygen that is 400 mL/min/mm Hg. During moderate exercise, the diffusing capacity for oxygen rises to 45 to 50 mL/min/mm Hg.

Factors Affecting Diffusing Capacity

- **Pressure gradient:** The partial pressure of oxygen is 159 mm Hg in the atmosphere and 104 mm Hg in the alveoli. Oxygen can easily enter the alveoli from atmospheric air because of the pressure gradient of 55 mm Hg. Similarly, the partial pressure of oxygen is 40 mm Hg in the pulmonary capillary. So the pressure gradient is 64 mm Hg between alveoli and pulmonary capillary which facilitates the diffusion of oxygen from alveoli into the blood. In the venous blood, the volume of oxygen is 14 mL% whereas in arterial blood it is 19 mL%. Thus, the diffusion of oxygen from alveoli to blood is 5 mL/100 mL of blood.

- **Solubility of gas in fluid medium:** If the solubility of a gas is more in the fluid medium, a large number of molecules are available for diffusion, resulting an increase in diffusing capacity. Therefore, the diffusing capacity is directly proportional to solubility of the gas.

CONSUMPTION OF OXYGEN

During exercise, the consumption of oxygen by the tissues, particularly the skeletal muscles, is greatly increased. Because of the vasodilatation in muscles during exercise, more amount of blood flows through the muscles. Therefore, more amount of oxygen is diffused from the blood into the muscles. It is well-known that the amount of oxygen utilized by the muscles is directly proportional to the amount of oxygen available.

OXYGEN DEBT

The term oxygen debt was coined by an English physiologist, AV Hill many years ago. It is defined as all postexercise oxygen consumption above the basal oxygen consumption level. In other words, it is the volume of oxygen used during exercise recovery above what is consumed at rest in the same period.

After a period of several muscular exercises, the oxygen requirement is more than the quantity available to the muscle. So the amount of oxygen consumption is enormously more. This extra amount of oxygen is required not only for the activity of muscles, but also for the reversal of some metabolic processes, viz.

- Reformation of glucose from lactic acid accumulation during exercise
- Resynthesis of ATP and creatine phosphate
- Restoration of amount of oxygen dissociation from hemoglobin and myoglobin.

A small oxygen debt can occur even in light exercise for which a steady-state can be aliened. Generally this oxygen debt is paid off quickly during the recovery period. During severe exercise, the oxygen debt continues to rise until the exercise ceases. The duration of the exercise is generally limited by the individual's ability to tolerate a large oxygen debt. An untrained sedentary individual usually stops work when oxygen debt reaches to about 10 L, whereas in well-trained persons, the debt capacity may raise upto around 17 to 18 L.

VO_2 MAX

The amount of oxygen consumed under maximal aerobic metabolism is called VO_2 max. It is the product of maximal cardiac output and maximum amount of oxygen consumed by the muscles. It is considered by most exercise physiologists, as the best single measure of cardiorespiratory capacity of an individual.

Table 5.1: Values of VO_2 max for male and female athletes of various sports events (after Shaver, 1981)

Events	Males	Females
Cross-country skiing	70 – 94	56 – 74
Long distance running	65 – 85	55 – 72
Rowing	58 – 75	41 – 58
Bicycling	55 – 70	–
Long distance swimming	48 – 68	45 – 60
Gymnastics	48 – 64	–
Speed skating	50 – 75	40 – 52
Ice hockey	50 – 60	–
Football	45 – 64	–
Sprints	–	38 – 52
Baseball	–	35 – 45
Tennis	42 – 56	–
Sedentary college students	45 – 53	30 – 44
Sedentary middle-aged persons	35 – 38	30 – 35

As VO_2 max is influenced greatly by body size, it is expressed in terms of milliliters of oxygen per kilogram of body weight per unit of time. It is reported that up to the ages of 10 to 15 years, there is very little difference in VO_2 max between boys and girls. However, for untrained adult college men, the average value of VO_2 max ranges between 45 to 53 mL/kg BW/min and for untrained adult college women, this value ranges between 30 to 44 mL/kg BW/min.

From Table 5.1 it is noted that the highest value for VO_2 recorded for a female to be 74 mL/kg BW/min for cross-country skier from Russia, while for a male the highest value was recorded as 94 mL/kg BW/min in the cross-country skier from Norway. It is also reported that, during exercise, there is an increase of VO_2 max by 50%.

RESPIRATORY QUOTIENT

It is the molar ratio of carbon dioxide production to oxygen consumption. When this is calculated under resting or steady conditions, it reflects the metabolic foodstuff being oxidized. The respiratory quotient is 1.0 one hour after meals. It varies with the degree of exercise. In moderate exercise, it varies from 0.85 to 0.89. If the exercise is prolonged with a high-fat diet, it falls to 0.7. But in severe exercise, the respiratory quotient value increases to 1.5 to 2.00. This is due to the greater hydrogen ion concentration in severe exercise than the moderate one being partly due to excess carbon dioxide and partly due to the entry of lactic acid from the muscles. Lactic acid combining with bicarbonates liberates more carbonic acid. In this case, respiration is much more stimulated and more carbon dioxide is liberated without any corresponding oxygen utilization, raising the respiratory quotient more than normal. In the recovery period, respiratory quotient falls to 0.5, because respiration is depressed and carbon dioxide is retained to form the lost bicarbonates. This carbon dioxide comes from the burning of the lactic acid part of Na^+ lactate in the tissues and combines with the Na^+ of the lactate, now left free.

NATURE OF SECOND WIND

During severe exercise, initially a frequent feeling of distress is developed. But if the exercise is further continued, this sense of distress is replaced by a sense of great relief. This is called second wind. The distress that precedes the second wind is:

- Breathlessness
- Throbbing of the head
- Fluttering and irregular pulse
- Muscle pains
- Chest tightness.

With the onset of second wind, the facial distress disappears and breathlessness other than discomforts disappears. The subject feels a sense of comfort. The second wind should not be confused with the steady-state which is the condition in which oxygen need and oxygen supply are balanced in such a way that the lactic acid and oxygen debt do not take place.

The physiological basis of second wind is not clear and it is a complex phenomenon in which different types of physiological adjustments take place.

ATHLETE'S LUNG

Athletes have more RBCs in their bodies, which make them more able to absorb oxygen in the lungs and move CO_2 out of the lungs.

They have stronger rib muscles which allow them to expand and contract the chest cavity more effectively and move more air per breath.

The increased chest size results in a larger number of alveoli in the lungs.

CHAPTER 6

Effects of Exercise on Endocrine System

In our body, numerous chemical reactions are going on. The endocrine affects bodily activities by releasing chemical messages called hormones, into the bloodstream from exocrine and endocrine glands. In fact, hormones are chemicals which cause certain changes in particular parts of the body. Homeostasis, i.e. equilibrium of the internal environment of the body is maintained partly by the autonomic nervous system and partly by the endocrine system. The autonomic nervous system is concerned with rapid changes, while hormones of the endocrine system are mainly involved in slower and more precise adjustments. They can control long-term changes such as rate of growth, rate of activity and sexual maturity.

The endocrine or ductless glands secrete their hormones directly into the bloodstream. The hormones are circulated all over the body and reach their target organs via the bloodstream. The endocrine system consists of a series of glands (Fig. 6.1), viz.

- The pituitary gland
- The thyroid gland
- The parathyroid glands
- The thymus gland
- The suprarenal or adrenal glands
- The gonads or sex glands
- Pancreas (both exocrine and endocrine gland).

THE PITUITARY GLAND

The pituitary gland is also known as hypophysis and is described as the leader of the endocrine orchestra. It consists of two lobes—(i) anterior and (ii) posterior. The anterior lobe secretes the following hormones:

- Growth hormone (GH) or somatotropic hormone (STH)
- Thyroid stimulating hormone (TSH) or thyrotropic hormone

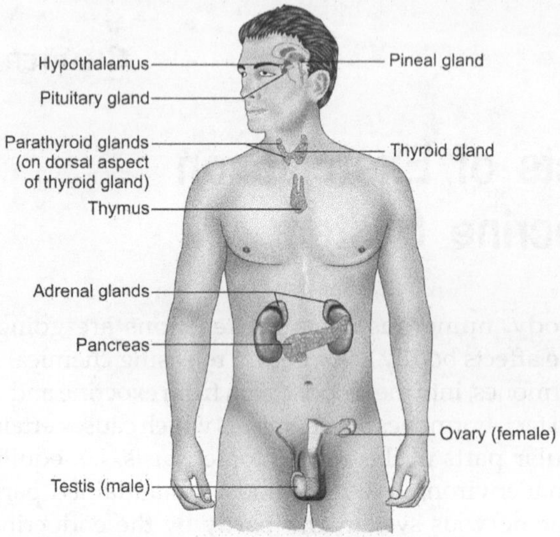

Fig. 6.1: Major endocrine glands of human

- Adrenocorticotropic hormone (ACTH)
- Follicle-stimulating hormone (FSH)
- Luteinizing hormone (LH in females), or interstitial cell stimulating hormone, (ICSH in males)
- Prolactin.

Growth Hormone (GH)

It is secreted by the acidophils of the anterior pituitary. Its release is stimulated by GH releasing hormone and inhibited by GH release inhibiting hormone (somatostatin), both secreted by the hypothalamus.

Functions

- It is responsible for the growth of almost all tissues of the body which are capable of growth. It actually increases the size and number of cells by increasing the mitotic division.
- It causes the specific differentiation of certain types of cells like bone cells and muscle cells. Thus, it is responsible for the general growth of the body. In children, its deficiency causes stunted growth leading to dwarfism. Its excessive secretion also causes enormous growth of the body leading to gigantism.

- It increases the growth of the skeleton. It increases both the length as well as thickness of the bones.
- It helps to increase the deposition of proteins by chondriocytes and estrogenic cells.
- It increases the multiplication of these cells.
- It increases the formation of new bones. This is because; the GH causes conversion of chondriocytes into estrogenic cells.
- It also acts on the metabolism of all the three major types of foodstuffs in the body, viz. (i) proteins, (ii) lipids, and (iii)carbohydrates.

Exercise Effects

In normal adults, the basal level of GH concentration in blood is upto 300 ng%, and in children it is about 500 ng%. The secretion is increased by exercise. Exercise of as little as 8 to 9 minutes in duration has the capacity to increase the concentration of GH levels (Mc Murry et al. 1991). This increment of concentrations of the GH is influenced by the intensity of exercise, duration of exercise, age, gender, and fitness levels of the exercisers.

Thyroid Stimulating Hormone (TSH)

This hormone is synthesized by the anterior lobe of the pituitary gland (Fig. 6.2). Its release is synthesized by thyroid releasing factor (TRF) from the hypothalamus. There is a circadian rhythmical release of TSH. It is the highest between 9 pm and 6 am, and the lowest between 4 and 7 pm. Secretion is also regulated by a negative feedback mechanism. When the blood level of thyroid hormones is high, secretion of TSH is reduced, and vice versa.

Functions

- It stimulates growth and activity of the thyroid gland which secretes the hormones thyroxine (T_4) and triiodothyronine (T_3).
- Thyroid gland secretes three hormones, these are:
  - Thyroxine (T_4)
  - Triiodothyronine (T_3)
  - Calcitonin.
- Thyroxine forms about 90% of the total secretion, while triiodothyronine is only 9 to 10%. Calcitonin is a calcium lowering hormone, secretes in a very less amount.

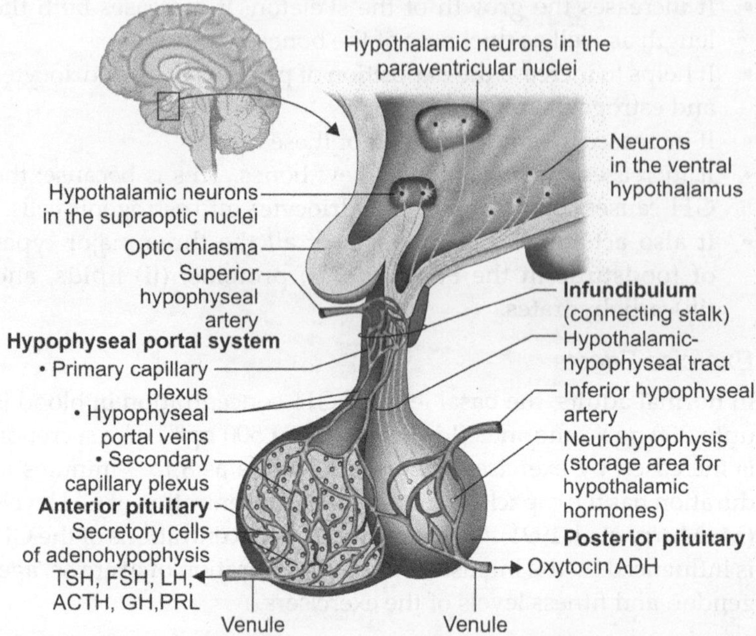

Fig. 6.2: Pituitary gland

Functions of thyroid hormones:

- Thyroxine and triiodothyronine are essential for normal body functioning by modulating metabolic rate and affecting glucose, fat and protein metabolism.
- Thyroid hormones increase oxidative metabolism in the mitochondria.
- These hormones increase tissue responsiveness to the catecholamines (Hedges et al. 1987).
- These hormones increase all aspects of lipid metabolism.
- High levels of thyroid hormones cause liver glycogenolysis and protein degradation.
- Low levels of thyroid hormones cause protein synthesis and conversion of glucose to glycogen. Thus, thyroid hormones aid in tissue growth and development.

Exercise Effects

Plasma TSH concentrations increase progressively during short-term exercise with increasing workload (Galbo et al. 1983). Galbo et al. (1983) and Wirth et al. (1981) stated that on short-term exercise, the concentrations of thyroxine and triiodothyronine and the clearances of this hormone were essentially unchanged.

Galbo et al. (1977) and Berchtold et al. (1978) found TSH concentrations to increase progressively with higher workload and to reach an elevated steady-state level after approximately 40 minutes of exercise. An increase of TSH might be expected to cause in increase in thyroxine and triiodothyronine, but physiologically the tissue is much more complicated with the thyroid hormones.

Adrenocorticotropic Hormone (ACTH)

This hormone is secreted from the anterior lobe of pituitary gland in response to corticotropin releasing hormone from the hypothalamus. The production of corticotropin releasing hormone is influenced by:

- Nerve impulses from the higher centers
- A low blood level of cortisol
- Physical stress, especially exercise
- Emotional stress
- Hypoglycemia
- Negative feedback mechanism stimulated by increased in blood ACTH and cortisol
- ACTH levels become the highest at about 8 am and fall to their lowest about midnight.

Functions

- It stimulates the flow of blood to the adrenal cortex.
- It increases the concentrations of cholesterol and steroids within the gland and increases the output of steroid hormones, especially cortisol.

Prolactin

This is a protein-based hormone released by the anterior pituitary gland. Its function is stimulated by thyroliberin and inhibited by dopamine. Both sexes can develop reproductive problems and disorders from excessive prolactin release. In women, oligomenorrhea and amenorrhea have been reported. Whereas, in men, oligospermia and testicular atrophy are associated with high levels of prolactin.

Functions

Prolactin is necessary for the final preparation of mammary glands for production and secretion of milk. Prolactin acts directly on the epithelial cells of mammary glands and causes localized alveolar hyperplasia which is essential for milk production.

In both males and females, release of prolactin is associated with a stress response. For this reason, it has been used as a marker of stress-reactivity in people.

Exercise Effect

With prolonged exercise, prolactin concentration increases, with the magnitude of the intensity of the activity (Galbo, 1983). With short-term exercise, the increase in prolactin may peak after the exercise bout if a steady-state has not been achieved (Poehlman et al. 1994). In some situations, excessive emotional stress can cause an increase even before the onset of exercise event (Hackney et al. 1989).

Gonadotropin Hormone

The gonadotropins are follicle-stimulating hormone (FSH) and luteinizing hormone (LH) which are released from the anterior lobe of pituitary gland after puberty in males and females. The glycoprotein-based gonadotropins are released in response to luteinizing hormone releasing hormone (LHRH), also known as gonadotropin releasing hormone (GnRH) from the hypothalamus.

Functions of FSH

- In females, it stimulates the development and ripening of the ovarian follicle.
- It stimulates the theca cells of graafian follicle and causes secretion of estrogen. As the level of estrogen increases in the blood so FSH secretion is reduced.
- In males, the FSH stimulates the epithelial tissue of the seminiferous tubules in the testes to produce spermatozoa in combination with testosterone.

Functions of LH

- In males, the hormone is known as interstitial cell stimulating hormone (ICSH) because it secretes the interstitial cells of Leydig in testis.
- This hormone is essential for the secretion of testosterone from Leydig cells. It stimulates the Leydig cells and the quantity of testosterone secreted is directly proportional to the amount of interstitial cell stimulating hormone available.

- In females, LH causes maturation of vascular follicle along with FSH.
- This is responsible for ovulation.
- This hormone is necessary for the formation of corpus luteum.
- LH activates the secretory functions of corpus luteum which secretes progesterone. As the level of progesterone in the blood increases, there is a gradual reduction in the production of the LH.

Exercise Effects

Research indicates that concentrations in the blood of the gonadal hormones may increase during short-term exercise, the increase being more pronounced the higher the workload (Raynaud et al. 1983; Hackney et al. 1997 and Galbo et al. 1989). These changes are probably due to decreased hepatic blood flow and clearance of the hormones.

The prolonged exercise-induced responses of the LH and FSH in the blood vary considerably for both men and women (Viru, 1992). Gender differences in the responsiveness of the gonadotropins may exist, in the form that the hypothalamic-pituitary-gonadal axis in women is a more sensitive regulating system than that in men (Hackney, 1992).

ADRENAL GLAND (FIG. 6.3)

Two adrenal or suprarenal glands are situated on the upper pole of each kidney. Each gland has two distinct parts—(i) the outer adrenal cortex and (ii) the inner adrenal medulla.

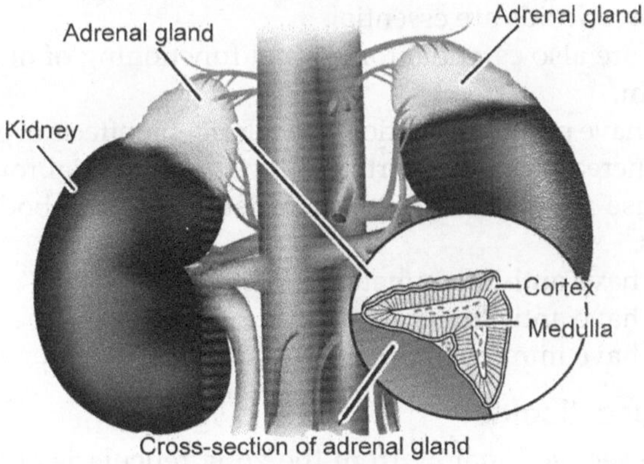

Fig. 6.3: Adrenal gland

- Hormones of adrenal cortex
- The hormones of adrenal cortex are also known as corticosteroids. These are:
  - Glucocorticoids
  - Mineralocorticoids
  - Gonadocorticoids

These hormones are mainly secreted from the zona fasciculata of adrenal cortex, though a small quantity is secreted from zona reticularis also.

Functions

- By promoting gluconeogenesis in liver from amino acids and by inhibiting glucose uptake and utilization by peripheral cells, glucocorticoids increase the blood glucose level.
- They cause catabolism of proteins.
- They cause mobilization and redistribution of fats.
- They enhance the retention of sodium and calcium (to some extent) and increase the excretion of potassium.
- Glucocorticoids accelerate the excretion of water when a large quantity of water is taken, causing maintenance of water balance.
- They increase the release of amino acids from muscle by catabolism of proteins.
- They decrease the number of circulating eosinophils by increasing the destruction of eosinophils in reticuloendothelial cells.
- For the constrictor action of adrenaline and noradrenaline, glucocorticoids are essential.
- They are also essential for normal functioning of our nervous system.
- They have permissive action like calorigenic effects of glucagons.
- The increase of glucocorticoid levels is essential for survival, because they offer increased resistance to the body against stress.
- They have anti-inflammatory effects.
- They have antiallergic actions.
- They have immunosuppressive effects.

Gonadocorticoids

They are secreted mainly from the zona reticularis and to some extent from zona fasciculata. Most of the hormones are male sex hormone (androgens). But small quantity of estrogen and progesterone are also secreted. The androgens secreted from the adrenal cortex are:

- Dehydroepiandrosterone
- Androstenedione
- Testosterone
- The adrenal cortex provides the only source of androgen in females.

Functions

- In general, the androgens are responsible for masculine features of the body.
- They are responsible for the development of male and female characteristics.

Exercise Responses

During short-term submaximal exercise, the secretion of ACTH is inferred from estimates of cortisol production. Galbo (1983) found no effect of low intensity exercise on ACTH secretion. But Kjaer et al. (1991) reported that two-legged knee-extensor static contractions at only 21% maximal voluntary contraction, stretched for 10 minutes caused an increase of ACTH concentrations. Barwich et al. (1980) reported a significant increase by 20 minutes of cycle exercise at 70% of VO_2 max. It is also reported that ACTH concentrations increase with the duration of dynamic exercise with intensity higher than 25% of VO_2max (Galbo, 1983). Ferrell et al. (1983) found that during moderate intensity exercise, ACTH levels increased about 10 to 15% as compared to 100% increase during high-intensity exercise and 400 to 500% increase during maximal intensity exhaustive exercise.

As cortisol release is under the influence of ACTH, at the onset of exercise, the release of this hormone is rather slow. But the levels increase proportionally with the increase of exercise intensity.

During intense prolonged exercise, the concentrations of ACTH increase drastically, resulting in significant release of cortisol (Galbo 1983 and Brooks et al. 1996). The magnitudes of the responses are modulated by both the relative intensity and duration of the exercise, the greater the intensity and the longer the duration the greater the release of the hormone.

Mineralocorticoids

They are secreted from the zona glomerulosa of adrenal cortex.

Functions

- They increase the reabsorption of sodium ions.
- They are responsible for the increase of volume of extracellular fluid.
- They cause persistent increase in extracellular fluid volume and blood volume which finally leads to increase in blood pressure.
- They increase the potassium excretion through the renal tubules.
- They reduce the hydrogen ion concentration in the extracellular fluid.
- They are responsible for the reabsorption of sodium from the sweat glands. The same effect is shown on saliva also.
- They are also responsible for the absorption of sodium in the intestines.

Exercise Effects

During exercise, the release of aldosterone (mineralocorticoids) is found to be partially dependent on the intensity (Fallo, 1993). Mountain et al. (1997) reported that 20 minutes of mild exercise caused the concentrations of aldosterone to increase by about 12%. Moderate exercise of the same duration results in about a 50% increase in aldosterone, whereas, higher intensity exercise results in about 75 to 80% increase. A high-intensity run at 80% maximal capacity until exhaustion caused a 10-fold increase in aldosterone reported by Melin et al. (1980).

Adrenal Medulla

It is the inner part of the adrenal gland. The active substances released by the medulla are the catecholamines:

- Adrenaline or epinephrine
- Noradrenaline or norepinephrine
- Dopamine.

Functions

Adrenaline increases oxygen consumption and removal of carbon dioxide.

- It increases the blood glucose level.
- It causes metabolism of free fatty acids from adipose tissue.
- It reduces blood coagulation time.
- It increases red blood cell count and hemoglobin content in blood.

- It increases overall activity of the heart, i.e. heart rate, force of contraction and excitability of heart muscle.
- Noradrenaline causes contraction of blood vessels throughout the body.
- Adrenaline increases systolic blood pressure but decreases diastolic blood pressure. While, noradrenaline increases diastolic blood pressure also slightly increases the systolic blood pressure.
- Adrenaline increases the rate and force of respiration.
- It increases the secretion of sweat.
- It causes the activity of brain. After exposure to stress, the release of adrenaline increases during fights or flight reactions.
- In brain, dopamine acts as a neurotransmitter.

Exercise Effects

The secretion of catecholamines is influenced by the intensity and duration of exercise. Kotchen et al. (1971), Christensen et al. (1979) and McMurry et al. (1987) reported that norepinephrine secretion was increased with the intensity of exercise. Even with low-intensity exercise, slight increase in secretion was evident. 20 minutes of exercise at 60% maximal capacity can increase double the circulating levels of norepinephrine and triple the levels of epinephrine.

With the increase of duration of exercise, the catecholamine output also increases. Kinderman et al. (1982) reported that 50 minute run at 60 to 70% maximal intensity resulted an increase of 300 to 400% in the release of epinephrine and 600 to 900% in norepinephrine.

PANCREAS (FIG. 6.4)

The endocrine function of pancreas is performed by the islets of Langerhans. Four types of cells are present in islets of Langerhans:

1. Alpha cells which secrete glucagons
2. Beta cells which secrete insulin
3. Delta cells which secrete somatostatin
4. PP cells which secrete pancreatic polypeptide.

Among these, insulin and glucagons are the important pancreatic hormones which regulate various metabolic processes of proteins, fats and carbohydrates.

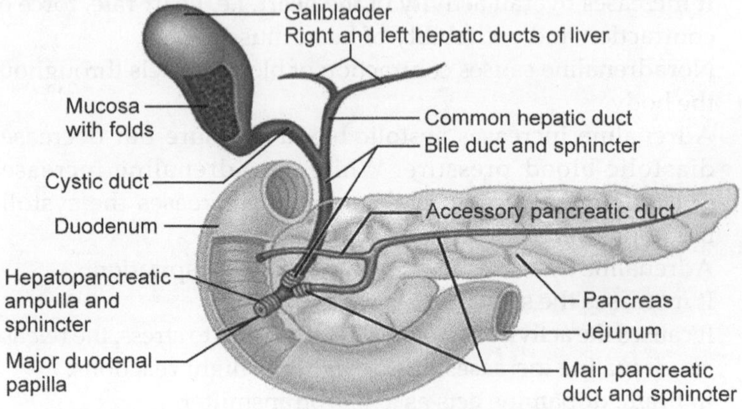

Fig. 6.4: Pancreas

Insulin

This hormone is synthesized in rough endoplasmic reticulum of beta cells in islets of Langerhans.

Functions

- When more carbohydrate is taken with food, the blood sugar level is increased. Immediately, pancreas secretes insulin which facilitates the transport of glucose from the blood into the cells by increasing the permeability of cell membrane to glucose.
- Under the influence of insulin, the peripheral utilization of glucose is increased.
- Insulin promotes the rapid conversion of glucose into glycogen (glycogenesis).
- Insulin prevents the breakdown of glycogen into glucose in muscles and liver.
- It prevents gluconeogenesis by inhibiting the release of amino acids from muscles and by inhibiting the activities of enzymes involved in gluconeogenesis.
- It facilitates the transport of amino acids into the cells from blood. It actually, increases the permeability of cell membrane for amino acids.
- It accelerates the synthesis of proteins.
- It inhibits the catabolism of proteins by inhibiting the activity of cellular enzymes which act on proteins.
- It causes synthesis of fat.

- It also causes storage of fat in the adipose tissue.
- It promotes growth of body along with GH.

Exercise Effects

The beta cells of islets of Langerhans have alpha-adrenergic receptors. Exercise elevates sympathetic activity which stimulates these alpha-adrenergic receptors, resulting decrease in insulin secretion. The effect was reported to occur even during short-term (10–30 minutes) submaximal exercise capacity (Gyntelberg et al. 1977; Winder et al. 1979 and Viru 1992), prolonged submaximal exercise of 60 to 180 minutes (Koivisto and Yki-Jarviner, 1987; Araujo-Vilar et al. 1997), maximal intensity exercise (Hartley et al., 1972) and even during resistance or strength exercise (Miller et al. 1984).

Felig and Wahren (1975) reported that the secretion of insulin decreased during exercise, but the cellular uptake of glucose could increase upto 20-fold. In fact, exercise increases blood flow, which supplies more glucose to the cells. Catecholamines in some way stimulate cellular uptake of glucose. The exercise directly stimulates translocation of GLUT4 transporters to the sarcolemma to enhance glucose uptake. All these factors may work synergistically to enhance muscle cell glucose uptake. The low levels of insulin permit mobilization of glucose from liver stores, fat use for energy, and gluconeogenesis, all necessary responses during prolonged exercise.

Glucagon

It is a polypeptide secreted from the alpha cells of islets of Langerhans.

Functions

- It increases glycogenolysis (breakdown of glycogen into glucose) in liver.
- It increases gluconeogenesis (formation of glucose from proteins) in liver by activating the enzymes which convert pyruvate into phosphoenol pyruvate and increase the transport of amino acids into the liver cells.
- It increases the release of free fatty acids from adipose tissue.
- It increases the secretion of bile.
- It inhibits the secretion of gastric juice.

Exercise Effects

It is reported that exercise has quite elementary effect on the release of glucagon. Short-term exercise of 13 to 15 minutes causes a small increase in glucagon release. Mild exercise at 40% maximal capacity for the durations of 40 to 120 minutes causes only 20% increase in glucagon release (Felig and Wahren, 1975 and Lavoie et al. 1997). Moderate intensity exercise (55–65% maximal capacity) for 90 minutes of duration causes 40–50% increase in glucagon release. Practically, alpha cells of the pancreas have beta-adrenergic receptors that respond to increasing epinephrine (Luyckx and Lefebvre, 1974). Exercise increases epinephrine concentrations which could serve as the initial stimulus for glucagon release. Researchers have also hypothesized that increased use of fats for energy during exercise may serve as stimulus for glucagon release (Jimenez et al. 1997). Moreover, decrease in insulin sensitizes liver cells to glucagon.

TESTOSTERONE

Male sex hormone is called androgens. Testis secretes three androgens:

1. Testosterone—It is secreted in large quantity by testes and in small quantity by adrenal cortex.
2. Dihydrotestosterone
3. Androstenedione.

Functions

After puberty, testosterone secretion causes increase in the size of penis, scrotum and the testis. Under the influence of testosterone, all these organs are enlarged at least 8-folds before the age of 20 years.

It causes the development of secondary sexual characteristics at puberty, distinguishing males from females. It helps in muscle growth, bone growth, change in skin, hair distribution and change in voice. Details are given in chapter 11.

Exercise Effects

During short-term exercise, the total and free testosterone levels increase which is proportional to the relative intensity of the work-load being performed. During prolonged exercise, testosterone responses are proportional to the intensity of the exercise, as higher intensities are performed testosterone levels increase. Details are given in chapter 11.

OVARIAN HORMONES

The female sex hormones, viz. estrogen and progesterone are secreted from ovaries.

Estrogen

Estrogen is secreted in large quantity by the ovaries and in small quantity by adrenal cortex.

Functions

- It causes the development of breast along with GH and thyroxine.
- It changes the vaginal epithelium from cuboidal into stratified type.
- It causes the enlargement of uterus.
- It increases the number and size of epithelial cells of fallopian tubes.
- It helps in development of hairs in the pubic region and axilla.
- It helps the larynx to remain in prepubetral stage which produces high pitch voice.

Details are given in chapter 11.

Progesterone

It is synthesized from acetate or cholesterol in the ovaries along with estrogen.

Functions

- It promotes the development of the lobules and alveoli of the breast.
- It promotes secretory changes in the uterine endometrium during the secretory phage of the menstrual cycle.
- It promotes secretory changes in the mucosal lining of the fallopian tubes. Details are given in chapter 11.

Exercise Effects

It is reported that 30 minutes of moderate exercise may increase the release of both estrogen and progesterone. Bonen et al. (1979) reported that 30 minutes of exercise at 70% maximal intensity may cause 38% increase in progesterone and 14% increase in estradiol release, but no change was occurred in the release of FSH and LH. The intensity of the exercise affects greatly to the increased secretions of estrogen and progesterone.

CHAPTER 7

Effects of Exercise on Nervous System

The nervous system controls all the important aspects of body function and maintains homeostasis. It controls and coordinates the functioning of all other systems in response to our surroundings. Each stimulus or change in our environment is detected by our senses and messages are interpreted by the brain which in turn, sends directions to the various organs to respond and adapt according to the external conditions which affect our body. The nervous system consists of the brain, the spinal cord and peripheral nerves. For descriptive purposes, it may be divided into three main groups, viz.

1. The central nervous system consisting of the brain and the spinal cord.
2. The peripheral nervous system consisting of the 31 pairs of spinal nerves. These nerves are divided into sensory, motor and mixed.
3. The autonomic nervous system consisting of 12 pairs of cranial nerves; some are sensory (afferent), some are motor (efferent) and some are mixed.

THE NEURON

The structural and functional unit of the nervous system is the neuron or nerve cell (Fig. 7.1). It is made up of three parts, viz.

1. Nerve cell body consisting of nucleus, Nissl bodies, neurofibrils, mitochondria, and Golgi apparatus.
2. Dendrites, the branched processes of the neuron have Nissl granules towards the nerve cell body.
3. Axon, the longer process of the nerve cell arises from axon hillock of the nerve cell body.

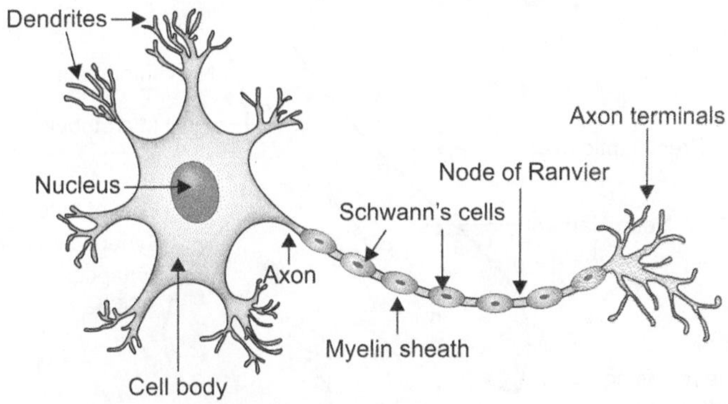

Fig. 7.1: Structure of neuron

Classification of Neuron

Depending upon the number of poles:

- Unipolar neurons
- Bipolar neurons
- Multipolar neurons.

Depending upon the function:

- Motor neurons or efferent nerve cells, which carry motor impulses from central nervous system to the peripheral effector organs, i.e. muscles.
- Sensory neurons or afferent nerve cells, which carry sensory impulses from periphery to the central nervous system.

Depending upon the length of axon:

- Golgi type I neurons having long axons.
- Golgi type II neurons having short axons.

SYNAPSE

It is a junction between two neurons, consisting of a minute gap across which impulses pass by diffusion of a neurotransmitter (Fig. 7.2).

Anatomical classification:

- Axosomatic synapse
- Axodendritic synapse
- Axoaxonic synapse.

Functional classification:

- Electrical synapse and chemical synapse.

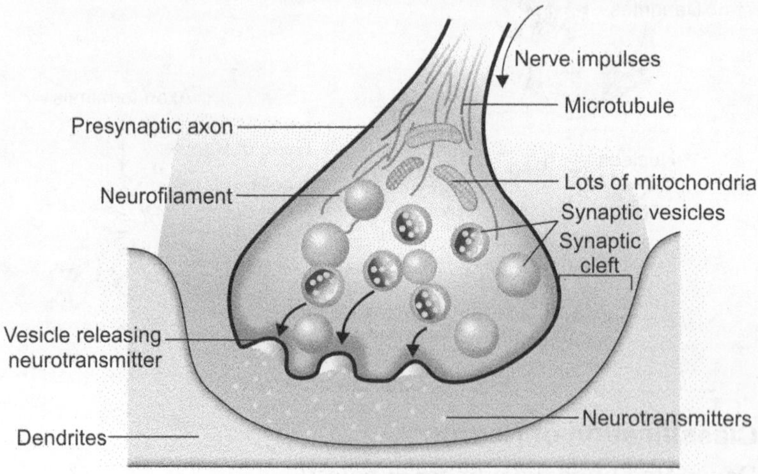

Fig. 7.2: Synapse

NEUROTRANSMITTERS

The chemical substance that acts as the mediator for the transmission of impulse from one neuron to another neuron through synapse is called the neurotransmitter. Some important neurotransmitters are:

Acetylcholine

It is the transmitter substance at the neuromuscular junction and possesses excitatory function. It is released also from various nerve endings, viz.

- Preganglionic parasympathetic nerve
- Postganglionic parasympathetic nerve
- Preganglionic sympathetic nerve
- Postganglionic sympathetic nerve
- Nerve in amacrine cells of retina
- Many regions of brain.

Noradrenaline

It is the neurotransmitter in adrenergic nerve fibers and possesses excitatory function. It is released from:

- Postganglionic sympathetic nerve endings
- Cerebral cortex
- Hypothalamus

- Basal ganglia
- Brainstem
- Locus coeruleus in pons, and
- Spinal cord.

Dopamine

The prolactin inhibitory hormone secreted by hypothalamus is considered to be dopamine and possesses inhibitory action. It is secreted by various nerve endings:

- Basal ganglia
- Hypothalamus
- Limbic system
- Neocortex
- Retina
- Small, intensely fluorescent cells in sympathetic ganglia.

Serotonin

It is an inhibitory substance which inhibits impulses of pain sensation in posterior gray horn of spinal cord. It causes depression of mood and sleep, vasoconstriction, platelet aggregation and smooth muscle contraction. It is secreted from:

- Hypothalamus
- Limbic system
- Cerebellum
- Dorsal raphe nucleus of midbrain
- Spinal cord
- Retina
- Gastrointestinal tract
- Lungs
- Platelets.

Histamine

It is an excitatory neurotransmitter. It is secreted from:

- Nerve endings of hypothalamus
- Limbic cortex and other parts of cerebral cortex
- Gastric mucosa
- Mast cells.

Gamma-Aminobutyric Acid (GABA)

It is an inhibitory neurotransmitter in synapses, particularly in central nervous system. It is secreted by the nerve endings of:

- Cerebral cortex
- Cerebellum
- Basal ganglia
- Spinal cord
- Retina.

Some other neurotransmitters are glycine, glutamate, aspirate, substance P, nitric oxide, etc.

Probably, the most important immediate response to physical effort is an increased activation of the sympathoadrenergic system. Nervous stimuli from the central nervous system to the adrenal medulla cause the hormone adrenaline to be released into the blood. Stimuli reaching the nerve endings in postganglionic sympathetic nerve fibers release the hormone noradrenaline. These two hormones have a number of different physiological effects, such as acting on beta-adrenergic receptors in the heart, noradrenaline and adrenaline increase the heart rate and the ventricular contractility (the strength of contraction at any given end-diastolic volume).

NEUROMUSCULAR JUNCTION

Skeletal muscle fibers are innervated by the motor nerves. Each nerve fiber divides into many terminal branches. Each terminal branch supplies one muscle fiber. The junction between the terminal branch of the nerve fiber and muscle fiber is called neuromuscular junction (Fig. 7.3).

The function of the neuromuscular junction is to transmit the impulses from the nerve to the muscle. When the impulses are transmitted from nerve to the muscle, a series of events take place in the neuromuscular junction:

- Release of acetylcholine
- Action of acetylcholine
- Development of end-plate potential
- Development of miniature end-plate potential
- Destruction of acetylcholine.

EFFECTS OF EXERCISE ON THE NERVOUS SYSTEM

Good coordination and balance is vital to the sports persons. The quicker the reactions, the more chance the individual has of having 'the edge' over the opposition, or of improving his or her personal best. As with most of the system, the nervous system can be

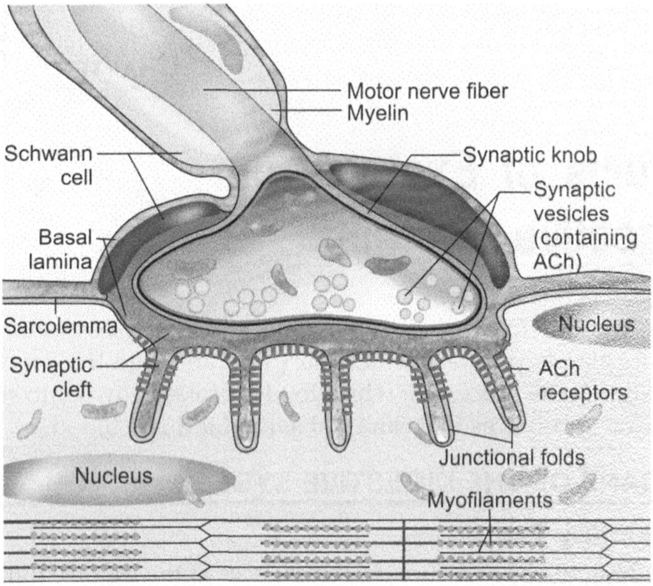

Fig. 7.3: Structure of neuromuscular junction

trained and improved with repetitive exercises. New and extended movements may be progressively attempted, practiced and perfected involving action through the use of the musculoskeletal systems and, as importantly, the voluntary nervous system to initiate those actions.

It is also important to realize that to some extent, nerves serving muscles under our conscious control work in pairs and therefore, when rehabilitating an injured part, it is often beneficial to exercise and stimulate the symmetrically uninjured part as well.

The nervous system is adversely affected by age. As we grow older, neurons are lost and not replaced. There is also a decreased capacity for transmitting impulses to and from the brain. In addition, both voluntary and reflex actions become slower.

The nervous system may be adversely affected by smoking, lack of sleep, poor diet, and stress.

CHAPTER 8

Effects of Exercise on Digestive System

Digestive system consists of alimentary canal, accessory organs, salivary glands, pancreas, liver, biliary tract and digestive processes. Digestion is the process by which food is broken down into simple chemical substances that can be absorbed into the blood.

ORGANS OF THE DIGESTIVE SYSTEM

Alimentary Tract

It is a long tube-like structure commences at the mouth, followed by pharynx, esophagus, stomach, small intestine, large intestine, rectum, and anal canal (Fig. 8.1).

Accessory Organs

Various secretions are opened into the alimentary tract:
Major salivary glands—3 pairs of salivary glands—(i) parotid glands, (ii) submaxillary or submandibular glands, and (iii) sublingual glands. Minor salivary glands—lingual mucous glands, lingual serous glands, buccal glands, labial glands, and palatal glands.
The walls of the alimentary tract: Four layers of tissue:

1. Adventitia (outer covering)
2. Muscular layer (muscularis propria)
3. Submucosa
4. Mucosa.

Functions of Stomach

- Temporary storage allowing time for the digestive enzymes, pepsins to act.
- Chemical digestion—pepsins convert proteins to polypeptides.
- Mechanical digestion—the three smooth muscle layers enable the stomach to act as a churn, gastric juice is added and the contents are liquefied to chyme.

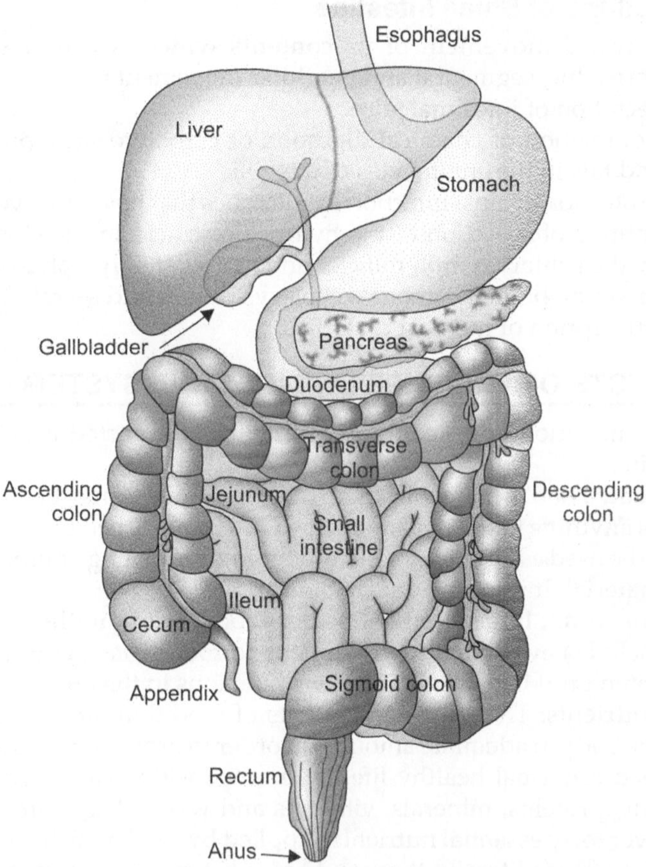

Fig. 8.1: Structure of digestive system

- Limited absorption of water, alcohol and some lipid-soluble drugs.
- Nonspecific defense against microbes is provided by hydrochloric acid in gastric juice.
- Dissolving out of iron from food—this takes place most effectively in the presence of hydrochloric acid although absorption occurs in the small intestine.
- Production of intrinsic factors needed for absorption of vitamin B_{12} in the terminal ileum.

Functions of Small Intestine

- Onward movement of its contents which is produced by peristaltic, segmental and pendular movements.
- Secretion of intestinal juice.
- Completion of chemical digestion of carbohydrates, proteins and fats in the enterocytes of the villi.
- Protection against infection by microbes that have survived the antimicrobial action of the hydrochloric acid in the stomach, by the solitary lymph follicles and aggregated lymph follicles.
- Secretion of the hormone—cholecystokinin and secretin.
- Absorption of nutrient materials.

EFFECTS OF EXERCISE ON DIGESTIVE SYSTEM

Food, nutrition and health are intimately connected aspects of our life.

- **Food:** Food is that which nourishes the body. It may be defined as anything eaten or drunk which can be absorbed by the body to be used as an energy source, building, regulating or protective material. It is a prerequisite of nutrition.
- **Nutrition:** It has been defined as food at work in the body. It includes everything that happens to food from the time it is eaten until it is used for various functions in the body.
- **Nutrients:** These are components of food that are needed by the body in adequate amounts in order to grow, reproduce and lead a normal healthy life. Nutrients include carbohydrates, fats, proteins, minerals, vitamins and water. There are about over forty essential nutrients supplied by food, which are used to produce literally thousands of substance necessary for life and physical fitness.

Energy

Energy is regarded as the capacity to do work.

- **Forms of energy:** There are five forms of energy that are relevant to exercise physiology. These are:
  - i. **Chemical energy:** It is stored or released during the making or breaking of molecular bonds.
  - ii. **Thermal energy:** It is absorbed or released in the form of heat.
  - iii. **Mechanical energy:** It is expanded in the performance of physical activities.

iv. **Electrical energy:** It reflects the work needed to move electrically charged particles against the forces produced by electric fields.
v. **Radiant energy:** It is transmitted in the form of electromagnetic waves.

Energy is used by the body for its various physiological purposes. The rate at which energy is used, varies greatly with different physical activities (Tables 8.1 and 8.2). Exercise increases this rate. In fact, it is the function of metabolism to provide this energy. Energy sources are stored, metabolized and utilized by the body. Food particles are ingested, absorbed and finally metabolized and transfer their chemical energy into high-energy phosphate bonds in adenosine triphosphate (ATP) which can be regarded as the energy currency of our body. During physical activities, the enzyme ATPase breaks the high-energy bond in ATP and makes the energy available for muscular contraction.

Table 8.1: Energy used in physical activities

Activity	Cal/kg/hr
Sitting and standing	1.7
Sedentary occupations (overall rate)	1.7
Light industrial work (overall rate)	2.5
Personal necessities, e.g. dressing, undressing, shaving, bathing, etc.	3.0
Walking (5 km/hr)	4.0
Active recreation (e.g. cricket)	4.0
Heavy work (overall rate)	5.0

Table 8.2: Recommended daily allowances for energy

Particulars of the individual	Calories/day
Man (55 kg)	
Sedentary work	2400
Moderate work	2800
Heavy work	3900
Woman (45 kg)	
Sedentary work	1900
Moderate work	2200
Heavy work	3000
Pregnancy (second half)	+ 300

Contd...

Contd...

Particulars of the individual	Calories/day
Lactation (up to 6 months) (7–12 months)	+ 550 + 400
Infants and children	
7–12 months	108/kg
4–6 years	1720
7–9 years	2050
10–12 years	2100
Girls	
10–12 years	2260
13–15 years	2360
16–18 years	2200
Boys	
10–12 years	2420
13–15 years	2660
16–18 years	2820

Sources of Energy

The major sources of energy in our body are carbohydrates, fats and proteins. They are provided by nutrients that must be digested and absorbed into the body.

- **Carbohydrates:** They are composed of carbon, hydrogen and oxygen molecules. They may be divided into:
  - **Monosaccharides:** It is the simplest form of carbohydrates that is not further digested. The main monosaccharides in the diet are glucose, fructose and galactose.
  - **Disaccharides:** They are formed when pairs of monosaccharides are linked together. The main disaccharides in the diet are sucrose, lactose and maltose. Sucrose is comprised of glucose plus fructose. Lactose is comprised of glucose plus galactose. And, maltose is comprised of glucose plus glucose.
  - **Polysaccharides:** They are large, complex molecules that consist of many units of monosaccharides linked together. Starch is a polysaccharide made by plant cell from units of glucose and glycogen is a polysaccharide made by animal cells from units of glucose.

DIGESTION OF CARBOHYDRATES

- **In the mouth:** The enzymes involved in the digestion of carbohydrates are known as amylolactic enzymes. The only amylolactic enzyme present in saliva is the salivary amylase or ptyalin. Ptyalin in saliva acts on cooked starch and converts it into maltose and a small quantity of glucose.
- **In the stomach:** The action of ptyalin is inactivated when the pH of the contents of stomach reaches to about 4. Thus, though the digestion of carbohydrates by ptyalin starts in mouth, it is completed only in the stomach.
- Gastric juice contains a weak amylase, which plays a minor role in digestion of carbohydrates.
- **In the intestine:** The carbohydrate splitting enzymes present in the small intestine are derived from the pancreatic juice and the intestinal secretion, succus entericus.
- Pancreatic juice contains pancreatic amylase. Almost all the starch is digested by pancreatic amylase within 15 to 30 minutes, after chyme enters the duodenum. Pancreatic amylase converts the starch into maltose, maltriose and dextrin.
- Carbohydrate splitting enzymes present in succus entericus are maltase, sucrase, lactase, dextrinase and trehalase. Maltase converts maltose and maltriose into glucose. Sucrase splits sucrose into glucose and fructose and lactase splits lactose into glucose and galactose. Dextrinase converts dextrin, maltose and maltriose into glucose. Trehalase or trehalose glucohydrolase acts on trehalose and converts it into glucose.

Absorption of Carbohydrate

The carbohydrates are absorbed from the small intestine mainly as the monosaccharides viz. glucose, galactose and fructose.

- **Glucose:** This is transported from the lumen of small intestine into the epithelial cells in the mucous membrane of small intestine by means of sodium counter transport. From the epithelial cells, glucose is absorbed in the portal vein by facilitated diffusion. Nonetheless, sodium ion moves laterally into the intercellular space. Then it is transported into body by active transport, utilizing the energy liberated by breakdown of ATP.
- **Galactose:** This is absorbed from the small intestine in the same mechanism as that of glucose.

- **Fructose:** This is absorbed into the blood by means of facilitated diffusion. Some molecules of fructose are converted into glucose.

Carbohydrate Metabolism and Exercise

This is the preferred fuel for the contraction of skeletal muscles during strenuous exercise. Since the endogenous carbohydrate stores are relatively limited, dietary carbohydrate intake is important for ensuring adequate carbohydrate availability before, during and after exercise.

Carbohydrate reserves: Ingested carbohydrate enters the bloodstream primarily as glucose. Carbohydrate is stored as glycogen. The liver has the highest concentration of glycogen (approximately 250 millimoles per Kg). But as skeletal muscle comprises about 40% of total body mass, this tissue contains the largest glycogen reserve.

The magnitude of both the liver and muscle glycogen reserves is very much influenced by the levels of exercise and dietary carbohydrate intake. Following a prolonged severe exercise, the liver can be completely emptied of glycogen, whereas, the liver glycogen can be as high as 500 millimoles per Kg following carbohydrate refeeding. Similarly, muscle glycogen levels may rise from close to zero to 200 millimoles per Kg, depending on the interactions among exercise intensity and duration, training status, and dietary carbohydrate intake.

Carbohydrate Metabolism Under Resting Conditions

Under resting conditions, the net muscle glycogen utilization is negligible and the muscle glycogen store is preserved for use during times of increased skeletal muscle activity. During and after exercise, the release of lactate from active and inactive skeletal muscles can provide a gluconeogenic precursor for the liver (Ahlborg and Felig, 1982 and 1986). The brain, central nervous system, blood cells and kidneys are dependent on glucose for energy supply. The liver glycogen store maintains the blood glucose levels between meals, ensuring adequate energy supply to these organs. Under resting conditions, these tissues account for about 75% of glucose utilization, whereas, skeletal muscle accounts for about 15 to 20%. At rest, glycogenolysis is responsible for about 75% of liver output.

Carbohydrate Metabolism During Exercise

During prolonged strenuous exercise, the energy is supplied to the contracting skeletal muscle through muscle glycogen and blood-borne glucose, derived from liver glycogenolysis and gluconeogenesis. Depletion of this carbohydrate release causes fatigue during such exercise (Coyle et al. 1986). Endurance exercise program is enhanced with the effects of increased muscle glycogen availability prior to exercise and carbohydrate ingestion during exercise (Coyle et al. 1986 and Hawley et al. 1997). This enhancement is due to maintenance of carbohydrate availability and oxidation during exercise. More has been discussed in chapter 9.

FATS

Fat is a major source of energy in the resting state and during prolonged low-intensity exercise. It is obtained mainly from the diet, but can also be synthesized in the body from carbohydrate. If excess fat is supplied in the diet, this may be stored as fat reserves in the body.

Functions

- They are the concentrated sources of energy.
- They are the carriers of fat-soluble vitamins and essential fatty acids. Details are given in chapter 9.

Digestion and Absorption of Fat

Fats are mainly digested in the small intestine with the help of bile salts and pancreatic lipolytic enzymes. Its different steps are:

- Emulsification: Entering into the small intestine from liver through bile, the fat molecules become water-soluble with the detergent action of bile salts. This action of bile salts is called emulsification. Emulsification divides fat into small droplets that present more surface area to digestive enzymes than do the original larger droplets, causing fat to mix with water, thereby forming a suspension.
- Pancreatic lipase is the most important enzyme for the digestion of fats, though the pancreatic lipase can digest only the emulsified fat molecules. It converts most of the triglycerides into free fatty acids and monoglycerides. Other lypolytic enzymes of pancreatic juice are cholesterol ester hydrolase, phospholipase A and B.

- Digested fat forms tiny particles with the bile called micelles. Micelles diffuse to the mucosal cells that from the inner surface of the intestine; the digested fat and most of the bile enter the intestinal mucosal cells. Intestinal cells incorporate dietary fat into larger particles comprised of fat and protein called chylomicrons. Chylomicrons are released into the general circulation so that absorbed fat enters the blood several hours after the fat is consumed.

Metabolism of Fat During Exercise

Fat represents a much greater potential source of energy quantitatively than carbohydrate. Each gram of fat provides more than twice the energy as the same amount of carbohydrate. Unlike carbohydrate, in the well-fed individuals, there is a virtually inexhaustible supply of fat in adipose tissue.

During light exercise, fat can provide most of the energy used by muscle. The fraction of the energy provided by fat varies with exercise intensity and duration as well as the state of training. For exercise, high-intensity exercise promotes carbohydrate metabolism, whereas, long-duration exercise promotes fat metabolism.

PROTEIN

During exercise, quantitatively, protein is a less important fuel than either carbohydrate or fat. Protein generally accounts for less than 2% of the fuel metabolism during exercise of less than one hour's duration; during prolonged exercise, protein can account for as much as 10% of the total energy usage.

Digestion

The enzymes responsible for digestion of protein are called proteolytic enzymes.

In stomach: Pepsin is the most important proteolytic enzyme of gastric juice. Optimum pH for the activity of pepsin is 2 to 3. The hydrochloric acid in the gastric juice provides the ideal pH for the activity of pepsin.

Pepsin acts on proteins and breaks them down into proteoses, peptones and large polypeptodes. So, the proteins reach the duodenum in these forms along with chime.

In small intestine: Most of the proteins are digested in the duodenum and jejunum by the proteolytic enzymes of the pancreatic juice and succus entericus. Pancreatic juice contains trypsin, chymotrypsin and carboxy-peptidases. Trypsin and chymotrypsin are called endopeptidases as these two enzymes break the interior bonds of the protein molecules.

Carboxy-peptidases from pancreatic juice break the terminal bonds of the protein molecules. So, it is called exopeptidase.

The final digestion of the proteins is by proteolytic enzymes present in the succus entericus. It contains dipeptidases, tripeptidases and polypeptidases. Pancreatic juice contains two more enzymes, namely, collagenase and elastase. Collagenase acts on collagen and elastase acts on elastic fibers.

Absorption

The proteins are absorbed in the form of amino acids from small intestine. The levoamino acids are actively absorbed by means of sodium cotransport, whereas the dextroamino acids are absorbed by means of facilitated diffusion. The absorption of amino acids is faster in duodenum and jejunum and slower in ileum.

Effects of Exercise on Protein Metabolism

Protein metabolism is influenced by exercise in two respects:

1. Protein catabolism is increased, releasing amino acids that can be used as fuel
2. Protein anabolism is increased, adding protein to muscle.

The former effect predominately during exercise of high intensity and/or long-duration, whereas the latter effect predominately during recovery. Therefore, although exercise promotes degradation of muscle protein and amino acid catabolism, regular exercise does not result in muscle atrophy in the well-fed individuals because protein synthesis is increased during the postexercise period. In addition, muscle protein content can be enhanced by appropriate training techniques coupled with appropriate nutritional support.

CHAPTER 9

Nutrition and Physical Performances

With the emergence of competitive sports, the question of what an athlete should eat to achieve his/her maximum performance is discussed. In Greece, during the 5th century BC, the practice of consuming large quantities of meat to replenish the supposed loss of muscle mass during heavy exercise, was reported first (Christophe and Mayer, 1958). Later, with the discovery of vitamins, the experimentations offered a new and promising dimensions based on the assumption that if a little of something is good, a great deal of it must be much better. Research findings have claimed over the last few decades that physical exercise performance can be significantly improved by special diets or dietary supplements (Fenn et al. 1983 and Karlsson, 1990).

CATEGORIES OF NUTRIENTS

The food components may be grouped into six different categories called nutrients. For the classification of nutrients, a food component must be digested, absorbed, transported through the blood, taken up into cells, and finally metabolized. Food substances that fail to meet all of these criteria are not considered to be nutrients, such as dietary fiber and some additives. The categories of nutrients are:

- Carbohydrates
- Fats
- Proteins
- Vitamins
- Minerals
- Water.

FACTORS AFFECTING NUTRIENT REQUIREMENTS

Numbers of factors are responsible for the actual amount of each nutrient that an individual requires. These factors include:

- **Genetics:** Genetic factors cause people to inherit different abilities to utilize nutrients or to recycle them.
- **Body weight:** The requirement for some nutrients is proportional to body weight, such as protein.
- **Age:** Age is one of the important considerations, as infants and children may need disproportionately more of a nutrient to meet the demands of tissue growth.
- **Energy expenditure:** Energy requirements differ greatly individual-to-individual so as the energy expenditure.
- **The composition of diet:** The composition of the diet is another relevant consideration. The recommended dietary allowances for nutrients involved in fuel usage—such as the vitamins, thiamin, riboflavin, and niacin depend on the number of calories that an individual consumes per day.
- **Physical state:** Physical state can also affect nutritional requirements. Physically fit person can take adequate diet regularly, with their maximum physical efficiency.
- **Occupation:** Persons those who are involved in sedentary lifestyle related occupation may consume less amount of nutrients than those who are involved in moderate to heavy physical labor.
- **Climate:** Energy expenditure as well as energy requirement of a person also vary in different climates. For instance, in hot climate, persons have a tendency to consume fewer nutrients. The opposite is true in cold climate.
- **Physical activity:** The most important factor is the physical activity of a person to consume proper dietary allowance. Persons involved in regular strenuous physical activities consume more nutrients than those involved in light physical work or sedentary lifestyle.

NUTRITIONAL SUPPORT OF EXERCISE PERFORMANCE

Long-term nutritional practice: It can influence athletic performance because an individual's diet can affect health as well as his / her body composition. For instance, deficiency of iron produces anemia, which could limit performance of an individual by reducing the oxygen content of his / her arterial blood.

Short-term nutritional practice: It can also influence athletic performance. For instance, during exercise, provision of fuels and fluids can improve endurance by replenishing dehydration.

Intensity of physical exercise: Increased physical activity raises total energy expenditure and therefore raises the dietary energy requirement. In some cases, athletes engaged in extreme activities (e.g. ultramarathons) may fail to eat adequate amounts of their normal diet to meet energy requirements during the event and could require high-energy supplements.

CARBOHYDRATE INTAKE

Carbohydrates are found in the diet in sugars, starches and dietary fibers. In fact, dietary fibers are not absorbed and so provide no energy value. Carbohydrates have several advantages compared with fats as the dietary sources:

- They are more rapidly absorbed.
- They maintain blood levels of glucose thereby sparing glycogen and protein from breakdown.
- They replenish glycogen stores in muscle and liver
- They are the only fuel that can be used by the glycolytic system.

HIGH CARBOHYDRATE DIETS

The diet where carbohydrates (in any form) contribute more than 50% of the total kcal is considered as high carbohydrate diet. If the energy intake of an individual is 2000 kcal, carbohydrate would be at least 1000 kcal, which is provided by 250 g of starch / sugar (carbohydrate yields 4 kcal/g) (Table 9.1). Athletes involved in endurance events may require much higher energy intakes.

Table 9.1: Carbohydrate content of foods

Food	G/100 g	G/unit	Calories/unit
Rice, rice flakes, semolina, vermicelli	75–78	19/25 g	86–88
Wheat flour (atta), jowar, ragi	69–72	17–18/25 g	82–87
Dals	58–60	15/25 g	84–87
Tapioca	38	19/50 g	80
Banana	27	22/80 g	95
Potato, colocasia, sapota, peas, jackfruit, yam	16–22	8–11/50 g	40–49
Mango	17	9/50 g	37
Orange, guava, pear,apple, carrot, onion, cluster beans	7–13	3–6/50 g	24–30

Contd...

Contd...

Food	G/100 g	G/unit	Calories/unit
Leafy and other vegetables	1–4	1–2/50 g	6–17
Milk	5	7 / 150 g	100
Sugar	100	5 / 5 g	20

EFFECTS OF DIETARY CARBOHYDRATE ON GLYCOGEN STORAGE

- For prolonged strenuous exercise, maintenance of muscle glycogen stores is essential. Dietary carbohydrate is necessary to replenish glycogen stores.
- Ingested carbohydrate is a source of blood glucose, from which glycogen is synthesized.
- Ingestion of carbohydrate increases insulin release too, which stimulates the pathway of glycogen synthesis.
- For these above reasons, high carbohydrate diets promote glycogen synthesis.
- Conversely, for rapid weight loss, intake of very low carbohydrate diets that are sometimes advocated popularly, leads to the depletion of glycogen stores in liver and muscle.
- Low levels of muscle glycogen diminish an individual's capacity to perform physical activities that rely heavily on glycogen stores, such as high-intensity exercises or long-duration exercises.

GLYCOGEN LOADING

The direct relationship between carbohydrate intake and glycogen storage is essential. The technique of glycogen loading or carbohydrate loading or super compensation is popularly used.

The underlying principle of carbohydrate loading is to deplete glycogen stores in the muscles that are most utilized in the activity and then to refill them with a greater amount of glycogen.

About a week before the event, the athlete consumes a low carbohydrate diet (e.g. 2 g of carbohydrate/Kg body weight) and performs high intensity exercise to exhaustion. A few days before the event, the athlete switches to a high carbohydrate diet (e.g. 10 g/kg) and dramatically reduces training intensity, in some cases, to no training on the day before the event.

Training is a necessary feature of this technique. Only those muscles that are trained during the regimen, exhibit enhancement of glycogen storage.

CARBOHYDRATE INTAKE BEFORE AND DURING EXERCISE

- Glycogen stores are depleted by fasting (including an overnight fast) and may therefore interfere the optimal performance of an individual. So a high carbohydrate meal should be eaten a few hours before an athletic event to replete glycogen stores.
- Within 30 minutes of the onset of physical activity, consumption of a high carbohydrate snack may diminish initial performance because of gastrointestinal distress or transient hypoglycemia, resulting glucose-stimulated insulin release.
- When the same amount of carbohydrate is consumed after the onset of exercise, hypoglycemia does not occur. Because the catecholamines that are released during exercise, suppress the release of insulin and therefore its effect on blood glucose.
- During exercise, muscle metabolizes glucose obtained from the breakdown of its glycogen stores and glucose that it takes up from the blood.
- Glucose is supplied to the blood by the liver through the breakdown of liver glycogen (glycogenolysis) and through the synthesis of glucose from noncarbohydrate sources (gluconeogenesis) as well as by the absorption of ingested carbohydrate from the gastrointestinal system.
- Thus, carbohydrate intake during exercise can mitigate the decline in blood glucose during prolonged activities and bring about a slower depletion of glycogen stores in liver and muscle.

POSTEXERCISE CARBOHYDRATE INTAKE

Carbohydrate intake is needed to replete liver and muscle glycogen stores. The period immediately after the exercise is optimal for glycogen synthesis, because:

- Blood flow and therefore glucose delivery of muscle is still high.
- Exercise-stimulated uptake of glucose is still high.
- The enzyme glycogen synthesis is more sensitive to insulin in the postexercise period than at other times.

For these reasons, the consumption of a given amount of glucose leads to the formation of more muscle glycogen in the postexercise state than in the resting state. Therefore, glycogen repletion is best served by the consumption of carbohydrate immediately after exercise.

FAT INTAKE

Fats are the most concentrated source of energy in our body. Each gram of fat supplies 9 calories. Storage of fat in adipose tissue does not require consumption of fat from the diet. Excess dietary carbohydrate can be converted to fat. It occurs during weight gain on high carbohydrate diets.

Functions

- Fats and oils are concentrated sources of energy.
- They carry fat-soluble vitamins, viz. A, D, E, K into the body and help in the absorption of these vitamins.
- They are the sources of essential fatty acids which are necessary for growth in the young and for the maintenance of a healthy skin.
- As fat is a poor conductor of heat, a layer beneath the skin helps to conserve body heat.
- Fat acts as a cushion to certain vital organs.
- The palatability and the satiety value of foods are greatly increased by fats.

Recommended Daily Allowance

In order to meet the essential fatty acid need, diet should contain at least 15 g of vegetable oil daily. To avoid complications resulting from excessive intake of fat, it is desirable to fix the upper limit of 30% of the total energy intake from fats and oils.

Sources of Fat (Table 9.2)

Vegetable cooking oils are extracted from oilseeds and nuts, such as groundnut, sesame or gingelly (til), mustard, sunflower and coconut. Butter and ghee are animal fats extracted from milk. Other animal fats are found in egg, meat and liver.

Table 9.2: Sources of fats

Food	g per 100 g	Calories per 199 g
Oil, vegetable cooking	100.0	900
Vanaspati	100.0	900
Ghee, cow's	99.5	895
Butter	81.0	729
Oilseeds and nuts	37.0-64.5	537-687

Contd...

Contd...

Food	g per 100 g	Calories per 199 g
Mutton, muscle	13.3	194
Egg, hen	13.3	173
Liver, sheep	7.5	150
Milk, cow	4.1	67

Protein Intake

Dietary protein provides amino acids for fuel and for building body protein. The amino acids that are made in adequate quantities in the body are called nonessential amino acids, and those that must be provided by the diet are called essential amino acids, such as leucine, isoleucine, valine, phenylalanine, tryptophan, methionine, histidine, lysine and threonine. Thus adequate intake of protein not only involves the total amount of protein but also the specific essential amino acids.

Functions

Proteins are responsible for building new tissues in growth stages of life, from conception upto adulthood, and after injury.

- They maintain the tissues, those are already built and replace the regular losses.
- They act as regulatory substances for internal water and acid-base balance.
- They act as precursors for enzymes, antibodies, and some hormones and one of the B vitamins.
- They are responsible for milk formation.
- They supply energy too.

Recommended Daily Allowance

The amount of protein required each day depends upon the quality of protein consumed. High-quality protein is used more efficiently. Protein requirements can be assessed by measuring the nitrogen balance of a person:

- **Positive nitrogen balance:** It is a condition in which nitrogen intake exceeds nitrogen output, indicating that there is a net addition of protein to the body. This occurs during childhood growth, body building, weight gain, and pregnancy.
- **Negative nitrogen balance:** It occurs when nitrogen output exceeds nitrogen intake or there is a net loss of protein from

the body. It occurs when weight is lost or when protein intake is inadequate.

- **Zero nitrogen balance:** It occurs when nitrogen balance is the usual state for healthy adults who are neither gaining nor losing weight.

Table 9.3: Sources of protein

Food	Protein, g/100 g edible portion	Protein, g/unit
Pulses, split and whole	17–28	4–7g/25 g
Nuts and oilseeds (except coconut)	16–32	4–8g/25 g
Milk	4	6g/150 g
Egg	13	6g/50 g
Fish, meat, poultry	15–26	5–8g/30 g
Cereals	6–13	1.5–3g/25 g
Vegetables, mature beans and peas	4–8	2–4g/50 g

The requirement of the body for protein as determined by nitrogen balance studies is between 0.5 to 0.6 g/kg BW in adults, when the source of protein supplies the amino acids in the proportion needed by the body. In practice, the recommended daily allowance for protein is set for 1.0 g/kg BW for adults.

Sources of Protein (Table 9.3)

Plants are the primary sources of protein, because they can synthesize protein by combining nitrogen and water from the soil, and carbon dioxide from the air. Among plants—pulses, whole and split, nuts and oilseeds, and in animals—milk, egg, fish, poultry, and meat are good sources of protein.

VITAMINS

Vitamins are organic compounds, necessary in the diet in trace amounts that have specific regulatory functions. Various functions of vitamins are:

They may supply the proteins of coenzymes that cannot be synthesized by the body.

- They may act as antioxidants.
- They may regulate gene expression in specific tissues.

- On the basis of their solubility, vitamins are conveniently classified into two groups, viz. (i) fat-soluble vitamins and (ii) water-soluble vitamins.

FAT-SOLUBLE VITAMINS

They can only be absorbed in the presence of fat. Therefore, the presence of some fat in the diet is essential for their absorption. Fat-soluble vitamins can be stored in the body and hence occasional intake of very high sources may help the body to tide over periods of low intake.

Vitamin A

Vitamin A was the first fat-soluble vitamin to be discovered. It is found only in animal foods, mainly as retinol. Though plants provide a source of vitamin A for animals in the form of carotenoids, the orange-yellow pigments. The chief source in human nutrition is beta-carotene, which the body converts to vitamin A in the intestinal mucosa during absorption.

Functions

Vitamin A has a number of different functions in our body:

- It is necessary for our normal growth and development. With the insufficient supply of vitamin A, the bones stop growing, before the soft tissues are affected.
- This may result in overcrowding of the brain and nervous system, cranial pressure and consequent brain and nerve injury.
- In some cases, the damage of the optic nerve may result in blindness.
- The deficiency of vitamin A may sometimes cause degeneration of nervous tissue without causing bone malformation.
- Vitamin A occurs in the retina of the eye. It is required in the process of vision to adjust to light of varying intensity. In combination with protein, it occurs in the light receptor cell in the retina. If the supply of vitamin A is inadequate, ability to adjust to changes in intensity of light is impaired, causing night blindness.
- The epithelial tissues cover the outer surface of the body, line the major cavities and all the tubular systems in the body. Inadequate supply of vitamin A may cause the suppression of the normal secretions and subsequently, produces a keratinized

(dry and horny) type of epithelium. The skin may become excessively dry and normal secretions of mucous membranes are impaired making them prone to bacterial invasion.

Recommended Daily Allowance

The daily requirement for vitamin A of an adult is in the order of 750 mcg retinol or 3000 mcg beta-carotene/day derived from foods of either animal or vegetable origin. The allowance for infants ranges from 300 to 400 mcg/day. As the child grows to adolescence, the need gradually increases. During pregnancy, no increased allowance is recommended, but during lactation, the allowance is increased to 1380 mcg retinol or 4600 mcg of beta-carotene.

Sources of Vitamin A

Vitamin A is present in animal foods only. The richest source of vitamin A is animal liver. Other sources are butter, ghee, milk, curds and egg yolk (Table 9.4). Apart from these, refined oils and vanaspati are also good sources of vitamin A.

Table 9.4: Vitamin A content of foods

Food	Vitamin A, mcg/100 g	Carotene, mcg/100 g
Liver, sheep	6690	–
Eggs	360	600
Butter, ghee (cow's)	600–960	–
Refined oil, vanaspati	750	–
Milk	48–52	6
Leaves		
Dark green, e.g. amaranth, radish, spinach	–	5000 or more
Light green, cabbage, lettuce	–	750–2000
Yellow or orange, vegetables and fruits, e.g. carrots, mango, papaya, orange	–	665–2740
Immature beans and peas, capsicum, tomato	–	80–595

Vitamin D

Sometimes vitamin D is called as 'sunshine vitamin', because, in the presence of sunlight, our body is able to convert a precursor present in the skin to vitamin D.

Functions

For the proper absorption of calcium and phosphorus from the digestive tract and their deposition in the bones, vitamin D is essential. So, formation of strong and rigid bones is not possible without the presence of this vitamin.

Recommended Daily Allowance

Dietary intake of vitamin D is not easy to determine. It varies also greatly person-to-person. About 200 International Units (IU) are reported to be the daily requirement of a child. In adults too, the daily requirements remain the same or may be slightly less in amount.

Sources of Vitamin D

The main source of vitamin D is the irradiation of the skin with sunlight. The midday sun is rich in ultraviolet light and helps in synthesizing this vitamin. Though fats are not good source of vitamin D, small quantities of this vitamin is found in liver, egg, milk and milk fat (butter and ghee), fish liver oils (such as halibut, cod, shark, sawfish, etc.).

Vitamin E

It has antioxidant properties and believed to prevent the oxidation of vitamin A and carotene in the digestive tract. It is also believed to regulate the rate of oxidation of foods inside the body. It is widely distributed in foods.

Vitamin K

It is essential for the formation of prothrombin in the liver. Lack of this vitamin prolongs clotting time and may result in excessive bleeding after an injury. Green leafy vegetables are the main dietary source of vitamin K.

WATER-SOLUBLE VITAMINS

Water-soluble vitamins such as vitamin B complex, vitamin C, are absorbed quickly in the body. The unutilized amounts of these vitamins are not stored in the body and excreted in the urine.

Vitamin B Complex

A number of substances are included in this group. Of these, three main vitamins, viz. (i) thiamin, (ii) riboflavin, and (iii) niacin will be discussed here.

Thiamine

Vitamin B_1 or thiamine was first isolated in 1926 from the rice polishing. It is also called as antineuritic or antiberiberi factor.

Functions

- It is necessary for catalyzing the oxidation of carbohydrates in the body.
- It helps in the normal functioning of the nervous system and the heart.
- It is essential for proper growth.

Table 9.5: Sources of thiamine

Food	Thiamine, mg/100 g	Thiamine, mg/unit
Pulses, oilseeds and nuts (except coconut)	0.24–1.00	0.12–0.50
Cereals		
Whole	0.20–0.98	0.05–0.24
Refined	0.06–0.12	0.01–0.03
Flesh foods		
Pork	0.54	0.27
Liver, sheep	0.36	0.18
Other flesh foods, eggs	0.03–0.18	0.01–0.09
Vegetables and fruits		
Fresh peas, beans, capsicum and seetaphal	0.25–0.55	0.12–0.27
All other vegetables and fruits	0.01–0.25	Less than 0.01–0.12
Milk	0.05	0.07

Recommended Daily Allowance

The daily allowance of thiamine is dependent on the total intake of calories, because it is involved in carbohydrate utilization. The recommended allowance of thiamine is 0.5 mg per 1000 calories.

Sources of Thiamine (Table 9.5)

Plant sources include pulses, nuts, oilseeds, and whole grain cereals. Parboiled rice and fresh peas are good sources of it. Green leafy vegetables and animal foods such as milk, egg, fish, and meat are also good sources of thiamine.

Riboflavin

Riboflavin or vitamin B_2 or lactoflavin or vitamin G is water-soluble yellow pigment. It is less soluble in water than thiamine and more stable to heat, especially in acid solutions.

Functions

- It is essential for the growth of our body.
- It combines with protein in the body to form a number of important enzymes related to several oxidation processes in the cell.

Recommended Daily Allowance

The recommended daily allowance varies from 0.7 mg for an infant to 1.7 mg for an adolescent. The average 0.6 mg of riboflavin per 1000 calories is recommended as the daily allowances.

Sources of Riboflavin (Table 9.6)

Milk and milk products (e.g. curds, milk powder, concentrated milk, etc.) are the rich sources of riboflavin. Liver and kidney of animals, pulses, green leafy vegetables, egg and meat contain a fair amount of riboflavin.

Table 9.6: Sources of riboflavin

Food	Riboflavin, mg/100 g	Riboflavin, mg/unit
Beal fruit	1.19	0.60
Liver, sheep	1.70	0.85
Dark green leafy vegetables	0.30–0.47	0.15–0.23
Milk	0.10–0.19	0.15–0.30
Pulses, whole and split	0.15–0.39	0.04–0.10
Nuts	0.19–0.97	0.05–0.24
Other flesh foods and eggs	0.09–0.44	0.04–0.22
Cereals and their products	0.03–0.29	Less than 0.01–0.07

Niacin

Niacin is also called as vitamin B_5 or nicotinic acid or pellagra preventing factor. It is very soluble in water and stable in air and not affected by heat, acid or alkali.

Functions

- It helps in the breakdown of glucose to produce energy.
- It acts as a component of an important coenzyme involved in respiration.

- It helps in normal growth of human body.
- It helps to stimulate the central nervous system.
- It acts as an antipellagra factor.

Recommended Daily Allowance

The daily requirement of niacin, on the basis of caloric requirement, ranges from 8 to 26 mg depending on the age and occupation of an individual. The daily recommended allowance is 6.6 mg per 1000 calories.

Sources of Niacin

Cereals are the major source of it, supplemented by pulses and meat (especially liver). Milk, egg, vegetables and fruits contain very small amounts of niacin.

VITAMIN C

Vitamin C is also called as ascorbic acid. The vitamin is a white, crystalline, odorless compound readily soluble in water. It is anti-scorbutic vitamin.

Functions

- It has immense contributions in immunity system in our body
- It helps to form erythrocytes and platelets in our blood
- It helps in the absorption of calcium and iron
- It helps to form fibroblasts and osteoblasts.

Recommended Daily Allowance

The recommended daily allowance is 20 to 40 mg for children and 40 mg for adults. For a nursing mother, an intake of 80 mg per day is recommended.

Sources of Vitamin C

Amla, oranges, sweet lime, grape-fruit and pomelo are excellent sources of vitamin C. Guava, cashew apple, drumsticks are also good sources of vitamin C (Table 9.7).

Table 9.7: Sources of vitamin C

Food	Vitamin C, mg / 100 g
Amla	600
Guava	210–310
Cashew fruits, drumstick leaves	180–200

Contd...

Contd...

Food	Vitamin C, mg / 100 g
Capsicum	137
Leafy vegetables	
Amaranth, coriander leaves, cabbage, radish tops, drumstick	100–150
Citrus fruits	30–63
Papaya, pineapple, tomato	25–55
Other vegetables and fruits	5–95

MINERALS

The mineral requirements are almost identical to that of general population. Nonetheless, as young athletes are in a growing stage, they require somewhat more dietary minerals than adults. The largest concentrations of minerals are in bones and teeth. Minerals are also found in soft tissues, such as nerves and muscles, in blood and other body fluids.

Generally the minerals calcium and iron are included in nutritional planning. The other major minerals present in our body are phosphorus, potassium, sulfur, sodium, chloride, magnesium. Others found traces are manganese, copper, iodine, cobalt, zinc, and fluorine.

Functions

- They maintain the acid-base balance.
- They maintain the water balance in our body.
- They help in contraction of muscles.
- They act on normal response of nerves to physiological stimulation.
- They help in clotting of blood.

Some of the minerals are discussed here.

CALCIUM

Calcium contains 2% of our body weight. Bones contain about 90% calcium in it. It is present in blood and lymph also.

Functions

Calcium is an essential part of all living cells. It is found in bones, teeth, in soft tissues and body fluids.

- It is involved in normal muscle contraction.
- It is involved in nerve stimulation.

- It helps in blood clotting.
- It helps in maintenance of permeability of cell membranes.

Recommended Daily Allowance (Table 9.8)

The ranges of allowance recommended per day are given as follows:

Table 9.8: Recommended daily allowance of calcium

Person	Calcium, g/day
0–12 months	0.5–0.6
1–9 years	0.4–0.5
10–15 years	0.6–0.7
16–18 years	0.5–0.6
Adults	0.4–0.5
Pregnancy	1.0
Lactation	1.0

Sources of Calcium (Table 9.9)

The milk of cows, buffaloes and goats is rich in calcium. Milk products, such as curd, paneer, mava (*khoya*) are good sources of it. Millets, ragi and sesame seeds (*til*) have a high concentration of calcium. Small fish (fresh as well as dried) is also very good source of it. Green leafy vegetables are also rich in calcium.

Table 9.9: Sources of calcium

Food	Calcium mg/100 g
Milk products	
Milk, fresh	120–210
Curd	149
Channa	208–480
Cheese	790
Khoya	650–990
Skimmed milk powder	1370
Whole milk powder	950
Fish, fresh	40–1600
Fish, dry	500–6000
Gingelly (sesame, til) seeds	1450
Ragi	344
Other nuts and seeds	230–300
Leaves, dark green	70–400

Contd...

Contd...

Food	Calcium mg/100 g
Pulses	60–150
Flesh foods, cereals	10–50

PHOSPHORUS

Phosphorus is also an essential part of living cells.

Functions

- It is necessary for building normal bones and teeth.
- It helps in maintaining an acid-base balance.
- It helps in the transfer of fatty acids.
- Phosphorus compounds are important cofactors in a number of processes, for example, energy metabolism.

Recommended Daily Allowance

For a growing child the recommended daily allowance of phosphorus is 1.5 g. For adults, the amount remains the same or slightly less.

Sources of Phosphorus

Cereals, peas, milk, egg, meat, fish (small sized) are good sources of phosphorus.

IRON

It is one of the important components of blood. 8–10 mg iron is found in 100 mL of blood.

Functions

- Iron combines with protein for the development of hemoglobin.
- It carries oxygen from lungs to the cells and carries back some of the carbon dioxide from cells to lungs.
- Iron is an essential constituent of many tissues such as blood, muscle, etc.
- It helps to regulate oxidation-reduction reactions in the body.

Recommended Daily Allowance (Table 9.10)

Table 9.10: The recommended daily allowance of iron

Person	Mg/day
Men	24
Women	32

Contd...

Contd...

Person	Mg/day
Pregnancy	40
Lactation	32
Infants	1 mg/kg
1–9 years	20–25
Boys 10–18 years	20–25
Boys 13–18 years	25
Girls 10–12 years	20–25
Girls 13–18 years	35

Sources of Iron (Table 9.11)

Egg, liver and meat contain iron. Among plant foods, cereals, whole wheat flour, rice flakes, leafy vegetables are good sources of iron. Pulses, treenuts, bajra, ragi, jowar are also very good sources of iron.

Table 9.11: Sources of iron

Foods	Iron, mg/100 g
Leafy vegetables, dark green	5–60
Italian millet, rice flakes, whole wheat flour	10–20
Rice, jowar, bajra, ragi	3–6
Pulses and treenuts	5–10
Flesh foods (liver, meat), eggs	2–6
Other vegetables	2–5
Fruits	1–3

WATER REQUIREMENT

Approximately 55 to 70% of the total body weight is made up of water. Healthy individuals generally require an intake of at least 2 liters of water per day in order to replace the water lost in urine, sweat, feces and expired air. Exercise increases heat production and therefore promote water loss through the production of sweat. Excessive sweat loss can lead to dehydration and higher sodium concentrations.

Functions

- Water is a universal solvent and is able to dissolve all the products of digestion.
- It is a constituent of all body fluids.

- It helps in the transport of the products of digestion to the appropriate organs.
- Blood contains 90% water and carries carbon dioxide to the lungs, nutrients to the cells and waste nitrogenous material and salt to the kidneys.
- Urine contains 97% water and has all the waste materials dissolved in it. Thus, body is able to excrete soluble waste products of metabolism.
- Water is required for many chemical changes to occur in the body. In the presence of water sugar is broken down to simpler substances.
- Water acts as a lubricant, preventing friction between moving parts of the body.
- Through the evaporation of water from the skin and lungs, the body temperature is regulated.

Daily Water Requirement

The amount of water required by an individual depends on many factors such as the environmental temperature, humidity, occupation, and diet. An athlete performing strenuous exercise may lose several liters of water and dissolved salts, thus needs replacement early. Generally an individual requires 1.5 to 2 liters of water per day.

Sources of Water

Water ingested as such is the main source in our body. Water is also consumed in our body with foods. Certain metabolic reactions carried on inside our body also release water. Water balance in our body is given in Table 9.12.

Table 9.12: Water balance in a healthy adult

Water intake	Water loss
Water intake 800–1100 mL	Urine 800–1000 mL
Water in food 600–900 mL	Feces 200 mL
Metabolic water 200 mL	Vapour 600 to 1000 mL (skin and lungs)
1600–2200 mL	1600–2200 mL

CHAPTER 10

Effects of Exercise on Excretory System

For the growth, activity and repair of tissues, energy is essential. When we take the food, it is digested and absorbed in the gastrointestinal tract. Then after absorption, it is transported to the tissues through blood. Likewise, oxygen is also transported from the lungs to the tissues through blood. With the help of oxygen, the food particles are metabolized and energy is released. At the same time, lot of waste materials and carbon dioxide are produced in the tissues. These unwanted waste products and carbon dioxide must be removed from our body to maintain homeostasis. Excretory system is a process by which these unwanted metabolic waste products are eliminated from the body.

Though in excretory system, lungs, skin, livers are engaged in the removal work of the excretory products of the body, kidneys are playing the major role in the excretion.

THE KIDNEYS

Kidneys are bean-shaped organs, about 11 cm long, 6 cm wide, 3 cm thick and weigh 125–170 g in case of males and 125–155 g in case of females. The kidneys lie on the posterior abdominal wall, one on each side of the vertebral column, behind the peritoneum and below the diaphragm. They extend from the level of the 12th thoracic vertebra to the 3rd lumbar vertebra. The right kidney is usually slightly lower than the left.

It has three layers, viz. (i) outer cortex, (ii) inner medulla, and (iii) renal sinus. On the medial border of kidney, there is a depression called hylum. Renal arteries, renal veins, nerves, and ureter pass through this hylum.

- **The nephron:** It is the structural and functional unit of kidney. Each kidney consists of 1 to 1.3 millions of nephrons. The nephron consists of renal corpuscle or Malpighian corpuscle and renal tubule.

- **Renal corpuscle:** It is a spheroidal and slightly flattened structure with a diameter of about 200 μ. It is formed by two parts—(i) glomerulus and (ii) bowman capsule.
- **Glomerulus:** It is a tuft of capillaries enclosed by Bowman capsule. It consists of glomerular capillaries interposed between afferent arteriole on one end and efferent arteriole on the other end. The blood pressure of the glomerulus is higher than in other capillaries because the diameter of the afferent arteriole is greater than that of the efferent arteriole. The walls of the glomerulus consist of a single layer of flattened epithelial cells.
- **Bowman capsule:** It is a capsular structure enclosing the glomerulus and formed by two layers—(i) inner visceral layer and, (ii) outer parietal layer.

FUNCTIONS OF KIDNEYS

Excretion of waste products: They excrete metabolic waste products; viz. urea, uric acid, creatinine, bilirubin, etc. heavy metals, drugs, pesticides, etc. are also removed from the body by the kidneys.

Maintenance of water balance: They maintain the water balance in the body by conserving water when it is decreased and excreting water when it is excess in the body (Fig. 10.1).

Maintenance of electrolyte balance: They maintain the electrolyte balance, especially sodium, with relation to water balance. When the osmolarity of body water is decreased kidneys retain the sodium, and when the osmolarity increases, they eliminate sodium.

Maintenance of acid-base balance: By eliminating certain metabolic acids, i.e. sulfuric and phosphoric acids, they prevent the acidosis and thus, maintain the acid-base balance.

Hemopoietic function: By secreting erythropoietin, they stimulate the production of erythrocytes. Erythropoietin is an essential stimulating factor for erythropoiesis. By secreting thrombopoietin, they also stimulate the production of thrombocytes.

Endocrine function: Apart from secreting erythropoietin and thrombopoietin, kidneys also secrete renin, 1,25-dihydroxy-cholecalciferol, prostaglandins for the body. They help in regulation of blood calcium level by activating 1,25-dihydroxycholecalciferol into vitamin D which is necessary for the absorption of calcium from intestine.

Regulation of blood pressure: Regulating the volume of extra-cellular fluid, kidneys help to regulate arterial blood pressure through renin–angiotensin mechanism.

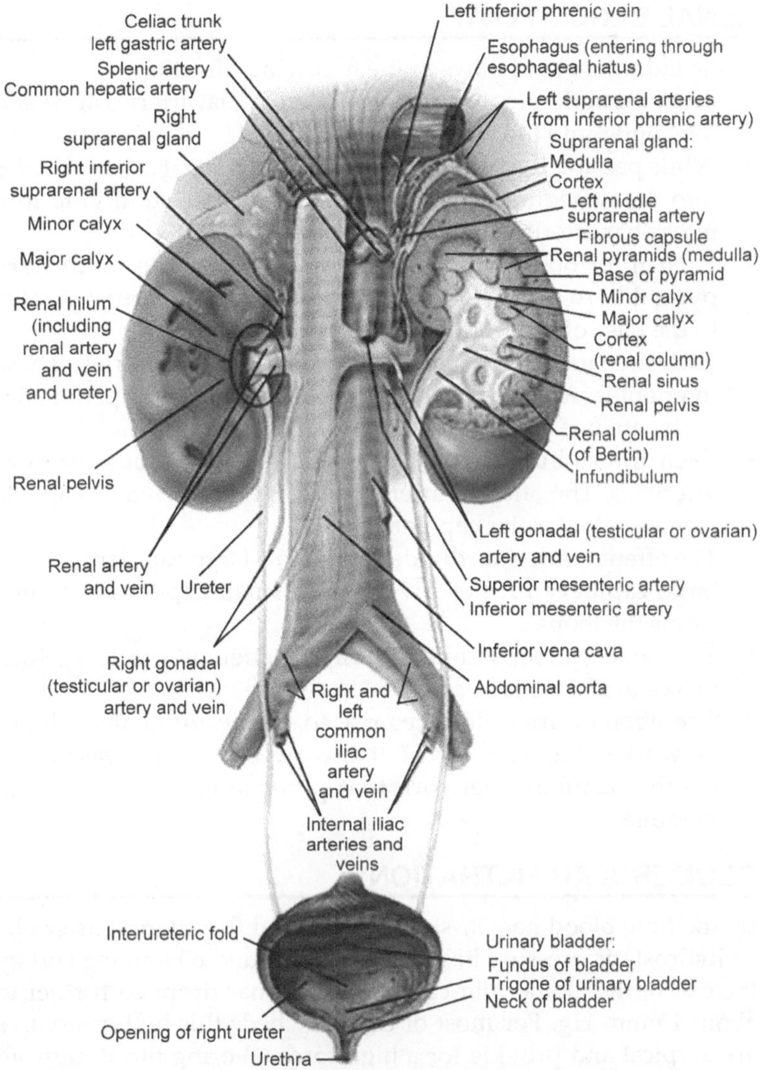

Fig. 10.1: Renal system of human

Regulation of vascular volume: During exercise, blood flow and oxygen consumption to the kidneys are decreased. In this process, kidneys play an important role in maintaining vascular volume.

RENAL BLOOD FLOW

In the kidneys, blood flows in the following direction:

- From the abdominal aorta, the bilateral renal arteries arise and then enter into the kidneys through hilus.
- While passing through the renal sinus, the renal artery divides into many segmental arteries which further subdivide into interlobar arteries.
- Each interlobar artery passes in between the medullary pyramids. At the base of the pyramid, it turns and runs parallel to the base of pyramid forming arcuate artery.
- Each arcuate artery gives rise to interlobular arteries. These interlobular arteries run through the renal cortex perpendicular to the arcuate artery.
- Each interlobular artery gives rise to numerous afferent arterioles. The afferent arteriole enters the Bowman's capsule forming glomerular capillary tuff.
- The afferent arteriole divides into 4 to 5 large capillaries. Each large capillary further divides into small capillaries, which forms the loops.
- The capillary loops unite to form the efferent arteriole which leaves the Bowman's capsule.
- The efferent arteriole gives rise to the peritubular capillary network in the renal cortex. It also gives rise to the vasa recta, another capillary network that plungs deep into the renal medulla.

GLOMERULAR FILTRATION

By the time blood has passed to the end of the afferent arteriole, its hydrostatic pressure has dropped to around 60 mm Hg and by the end of the glomerular capillary bed it has dropped further to about 15 mm Hg. For most of capillary beds this high pressures are atypical and provide for a high force favoring filtration from the blood into the urinary space. Because the hydrostatic pressure drops some 45 mm Hg across the glomerular capillaries, forces favoring filtration from the blood are stronger at the beginning of the glomerular capillary bed.

Colloid osmotic pressure is primarily a function of the protein content of the blood. Because proteins are large molecular weight substances, they do not pass readily through the glomerular membrane. Colloid osmotic pressures at the beginning of the glomerulus are about 28 mm Hg and have increased to about 36 mm Hg by the end of the glomerulus because of loss of fluid into the urinary space. The combined effects of hydrostatic pressure and colloid osmotic pressure favor filtration at the beginning of the glomerulus (by about 28-60 mm Hg or 32 mm Hg in average) and reabsorption at the end of the glomerulus (by about 15-36 mm Hg or 21 mm Hg in average).

HORMONAL EFFECTS ON URINE COMPOSITION

Aldosterone

It is a mineralocorticoid hormone secreted from the adrenal medulla. During exercise, the concentration of this hormone increases. The primary stimuli to aldosterone release are angiotensin-II and high levels of potassium. Aldosterone acts on the distal tubule of the nephron and promotes the exchange of sodium for potassium. Since sodium is the primary osmole of the extracellular fluid, its retention by the kidneys helps to maintain water volume in the vascular space.

Vasopressin

It is produced by the posterior pituitary gland in response to increased osmolality of the blood and decreased blood pressure. The decrease in urine volume produced by vasopressin is rapid, and it exerts its effect by increasing the permeability of water to the cells of the collecting duct. Without vasopressin, these cells are normally impermeable to water, but in its presence they allow water to follow its osmotic pressure gradient into the renal medulla. The net effect is that a more concentrated urine is produced when blood volume is reduced or its osmotic concentration is increased.

Renin

The granular cells (juxtaglomerular cells) of juxtaglomerular apparatus secrete the hormone renin. Renin is a glycoprotein with 340 amino acids. When renin is released into the blood, it acts on a specific plasma protein called angiotensinogen (renin substrate). It is an alpha-2 globulin. By the activity of renin, the angiotensinogen is converted into a decapeptide called angiotensin—I. This is further converted into angiotensin, II. It has three actions:

1. It causes constriction of systemic arterioles leading to elevation of blood pressure.
2. It stimulates the adrenal cortex to secrete aldosterone. Aldosterone acts on kidneys resulting in sodium retention.
3. It helps to maintain the glomerular filtration rate.

Regulation of Renin Secretion

Secretion of renin is stimulated by five factors:

1. Fall in arterial blood pressure.
2. Reduction in the volume of extracellular fluid.
3. Increased sympathetic activity.
4. Decreased load of sodium and chloride in macula densa.
5. Direct stimulation of beta-receptors on the juxtaglomerular cells.

Erythropoietin

Peritubular capillaries in the kidneys secrete erythropoietin. It is secreted whenever there is hypoxic condition. It is a glycoprotein with 165 amino acids. Erythropoietin stimulates the bone marrow and causes formation and release of new red blood cells into circulation. After secretion, it takes 4 to 5 days to show the action. The hormone promotes the following processes:

- Production of proerythroblasts from the stem cells in CFU-E of the bone marrow.
- Development of proerythroblasts into matured red blood cells through the normoblastic stages—early, intermediate and late normoblasts, and reticulocyte.
- Release of matured erythrocytes into blood through the capillary membrane from bone marrow.

Any form of chronic hypoxia increases the production of erythropoietin by the kidneys. Typically, athletes travel to high altitudes (more than 5000 feet) to stimulate its production but the increase in red blood cell mass that results, takes at least 5 days.

CHAPTER 11

Effects of Exercise on Reproductive System

Gender differences in body structure and function affect the physical performance of an individual. Some sex hormones are responsible for growth and reproductive maturation of human. Exercise has a strong impact with the secretion of reproductive hormones. For this reason, these hormones are sometimes manipulated by some sports persons in attempts to enhance performance.

REPRODUCTIVE HORMONES AND EXERCISE

Male sex hormones are called androgens. Testis secretes three androgens, these are:

1. Testosterone
2. Dihydrotestosterone
3. Androstenedione

Testosterone is secreted in large quantities while dihydrotestosterone is more active.

TESTOSTERONE

Testosterone is the major male sex hormone. In males, hormones from the hypothalamus and anterior pituitary give signal for the production of testosterone. Specifically, low circulating testosterone feeds back to cause the release of gonadotropin-releasing hormone (GnRH) from the hypothalamus. The gonadotropin-releasing hormone stimulates the release of follicle stimulating hormone and luteinizing hormone from the anterior pituitary. The luteinizing hormone in turn stimulates the cells of Leydig in the testis to produce and release testosterone. In males, this interaction of hormones and glands is referred to as the hypothalamic-pituitary-gonadal axis (Hackney, 1996). For females, testosterone is released primarily from the adrenal cortex through a mechanism that also implements the release of the glucocorticoids and / or mineralocorticoids (i.e. the hypothalamic-pituitary-adrenal axis). Physiologically, testosterone, a steroid-based hormone, has both anabolic and androgenic effects in each sex and is considered essential for proper growth, development, sex differentiation, and reproductive function.

Functions

- At the 7th week of intrauterine life, the presence of testosterone differentiates the sex by developing male sex organs from wolffian duct and by disappearing Müllerian duct.
- In fetal life, it is essential for the growth of the external genitalia – penis and scrotum and other accessory sex organs—epididymis, vas deferens and seminal vesicles, and prostate.
- Initially, testes are developed in the abdominal cavity and just before birth, they are pushed into the scrotum through inguinal canal. The process by which testes enter the scrotum is called the descent of testes. Testosterone is responsible for this descent of testes.
- After puberty, the testosterone secretion causes increase in the size of penis, scrotum and the testes.
- After puberty, one of the most important male sexual characters is the development of musculature. The acceleration of transport of amino acid into muscle cells, synthesis and storage of proteins, and considerable increment of muscle mass occur due to the anabolic activity of testosterone on proteins.
- After puberty, the bones grow in thickness. The thickness of bones is associated with deposition of calcium on it. Moreover, the increase in thickness is due to increase in total content of bone matrix. The anabolic activity of testosterone on protein may cause the increase in bone matrix. Nonetheless, testosterone causes broadening of shoulders, narrowing of pelvic outlet, lengthening and funnel-like shape of penis.
- Testosterone increases the basal metabolic rate to about 5 to 10% at the time of adolescence due to its anabolic effects on protein metabolism.
- It increases the retention of sodium by reabsorption in renal tubules, subsequently increasing the volume of extracellular fluid.

- After puberty, testosterone causes mild increase in blood volume by increasing the water content and by increasing the number of red blood cells.
- Due to the deposition of proteins in skin, testosterone increases the thickness of it over the entire body surface and the ruggedness of subcutaneous tissue.
- It also enhances the secretory activity of sebaceous glands.
- It causes male type of distribution of hair on the body, i.e. hair growth over the pubis, along linea alba upto umbilicus, on face, on chest and other parts of the body like back.
- At puberty, testosterone is responsible for the hypertrophy of laryngeal muscles, enlargement of larynx and lengthening, and thickening of vocal cords, producing a typical adult male voice.

Exercise Effects

During short-term exercise:

- The total and free testosterone levels increase.
- This increase is proportional to the relative intensity of performed workload (Sutton et al. 1973; Galbo, 1983; Hackney et al. 1990 and Poehlman, 1994).
- This increase is due to a decrease in metabolic clearance rate (MCR), an increase in secretion production and exercise-induced hemoconcentration (Hackney, 1996).

During prolonged exercise:

- Testosterone concentrations are either increased or decreased (Viru, 1992 and Jimenz et al. 1997).
- When exercise with higher intensity is performed, testosterone levels increase.
- When duration of exercise bout is longer (60–90 minutes or more), testosterone levels start to decline.

During maximal exercise:

- Testosterone levels are increased significantly (Sutton, 1973 and Galbo et al. 1977) due to hemoconcentration, decreased metabolic clearance rate and catecholamine-stimulated gonadal secretion production (Hackney, 1989).

After resistance-based exercise:

- Depending upon the intensity of exercise, volume of exercise, amount of muscle tissue used in the exercise protocol and age of the subject, the testosterone levels are increased (Kreamer, 1988; Passelegue et al. 1995 and McMurray et al. 1995).

OVARIAN HORMONES

Ovary secretes two important female sex hormones, viz. (i) estrogen and (ii) progesterone. Ovaries also secrete small quantities of androgens and relaxin.

Estrogen

In a normal nonpregnant female, estrogen is secreted in large quantity by the ovaries though adrenal cortex also secretes small quantities of estrogen. In pregnancy, a large amount of estrogen is secreted by placenta.

Functions

Estrogen causes the enlargement of uterus with the help of increase in size of the endometrial cells.

- It causes proliferation of the endometrial stroma.
- Estrogen increases the blood supply to endometrium.
- It helps in deposition of glycogen and fats in the endometrium.
- It helps in proliferation and dilatation of blood vessels of endometrial glands which become more tortuous with increased blood flow.
- It increases the spontaneous activity of the uterine muscles and sensitivity of oxytocin.
- It increases the actomyosin contraction causing the increase in the contractility of the uterine muscles.
- Estrogen acts on the mucosal lining of the fallopian tubes and increases the number and size of the epithelial cells, especially the ciliated epithelial cells lining the fallopian tubes.
- It increases the activity of the cilia, so that the movement of the ovum in the fallopian tube is facilitated.
- Estrogen also enhances the proliferation of glandular tissues in fallopian tubes.
- At puberty, estrogen is responsible for the development of the stromal tissues of the breasts.
- It causes the growth of an extensive ductile system in the breasts.
- It helps for the deposition of fat in the ductile system.
- Estrogen changes the vaginal epithelium from cuboidal into stratified type. The stratified epithelium is more resistant to trauma and infection.
- It increases the layers of the vaginal epithelium by proliferation.
- It increases the pH of the vagina causing more acidity.

- Estrogen is responsible for the development of hair in the pubic region and axilla.
- Estrogen renders softness and smoothness of the skin.
- The vascularity of the skin is also increased with the effect of estrogen.
- With the influence of estrogen, the shoulders become narrow, hip broadens, the thighs converge, and the arms diverge. The fat deposition also increases in the breasts and buttocks.
- By the influence of estrogen, the larynx remains in prepubertal stage, producing high-pitched voice.
- At the time of puberty, estrogen increases osteoblastic activity, resulting the enormous increment of growth rate of bones. But at the same time, estrogen causes early fusion of the epiphysis with the shafts, resulting early cessation of growth in females than males.
- In old age, due to lack of adequate secretion of estrogen, osteoporosis occurs.
- Estrogen induces anabolism of proteins, promoting the growth of the sexual organs, bones and a few other tissues of the body.
- Estrogen causes the deposition of fat on the subcutaneous tissues, breasts, buttocks and thighs, resulting the lesser specific gravity of the female body than that of males.
- Estrogen causes the retention of sodium and water by the renal tubules.

Progesterone

A small quantity of progesterone is secreted by the ovaries during the follicular stage of menstrual cycle. But a large quantity of progesterone is secreted during the secretory phase by the corpus luteum. Adrenal cortex also secretes a small quantity of progesterone. During the first trimester of pregnancy, a large quantity of progesterone is secreted by the corpus luteum. But in the second and third trimesters, placenta secretes large quantity of progesterone.

Functions

Progesterone increases the thickness of the endometrium by increasing the number and size of the cells.

- It increases the size of the uterine glands.
- It increases the secretory activities of glandular epithelial cells of uterus.

- It increases the deposition of lipid and glycogen in the stromal cells of the breasts.
- With the increase of size of the vessels and vasodilatation, progesterone increases the blood supply to endometrium.
- It decreases the frequency of uterine contractions, preventing the expulsion of the implanted ovum.
- Progesterone promotes secretory changes in the mucosal lining of the fallopian tubules.
- By proliferating and enlarging the alveolar cells, it promotes the development of the lobules and alveoli of the breasts.
- By increasing the secretory activity and fluid accumulation in the subcutaneous tissue, it makes the breasts secretory in nature.
- Progesterone increases reabsorption of sodium and water through the renal tubules.

Exercise Effects

- 30 minutes of exercise at 70% maximal intensity causes 38% increase in progesterone and 14% increase in estradiol secretions (Bonen et al. 1979).
- Same duration of exercise does not change the concentrations of follicle stimulating hormone and luteinizing hormone.
- When the intensity of exercise is increased, the secretion of progesterone is also increased, but the result is not consistent with estrogen (Jurkowski et al. 1978).
- During short-term and prolonged submaximal exercise, the secretion of progesterone and estrogen hormones is also increased (Bullen et al. 1984 and Keizer et al. 1987).
- Exercise during luteal phase of menstrual cycle, causes 40% increase in case of progesterone and 21% increase in case of estradiol (Bonen et al. 1979).
- Chronic exercise or exercise training decreases the resting levels of estrogen and progesterone (Bonen et al. 1981; Bullen et al. 1984 and Keizer and Rogol, 1990).

The more prolonged and intensed exercise sometimes causes the risk of menstrual irregularities and amenorrhea or loses of menstrual cycle (Elias and Wilson, 1993) in athletes. Exercise causes an increase in beta-endorphin which blocks the release of gonadotropin-releasing factor from the hypothalamus. Thus, reduced gonadotropin-releasing factor suppresses luteinizing hormone and follicle stimulating hormone, resulting in low estrogen and progesterone secretion.

CHAPTER 12

Temperature Regulation

Human is the most adjustable animal in the Earth. The protected human being can tolerate variations in environmental temperature between – 50°C and 100°C. But a person can tolerate a variation of only about 4° in deep body temperature with impairment of optimal physical and mental performance. Changes in body temperature affect cellular structure, enzyme actions and various chemical reactions in the body. The prevailing level of body temperature reflects a balance between the rate at which heat is added to the body and the rate at which heat is removed from the body. Body temperature rises when heat gain exceeds heat loss and falls when heat loss exceeds heat gain.

We know that under normal conditions, the internal temperature of our body generally remains at a constant level of 37°C. Temperature at different parts of body are axillary temperature is slightly lower (about 0.37°C or 1°F) than the oral temperature, rectal temperature is slightly higher (about 0.37°C or 1°F) than the oral temperature. The superficial temperature (skin or surface temperature) caries between 29.5°C (85°F) and 33.9°C (93°F), the core temperature is always more than oral temperature. In fact the core temperature is 36.8°C.

Several factors such as exercise, illness and external temperature may alter this consistency by either increasing or decreasing the body temperature. The neural and hormonal mechanisms cause the body to gain heat when core temperature falls below 37°C, as can occur in a cold environment, and to lose heat when core temperature rises above 37°C, as can occur during vigorous exercise.

HEAT PRODUCTION

Heat is gained by our body due to the combined effects of heat production by the internal metabolic processes of the body and external heat absorption from the environment by radiation and convection, such as the sun, a newly resurfaced black-top road, desert sand and rock, etc. if their temperature is higher than the body. The heat produced by the body is a by- product of chemical reactions that transform bond energy into work and heat. In fact, heat production from metabolism takes place in the tissues. Albeit, all tissues contribute to this, the skeletal muscles produce the largest amount of heat. Therefore, heat production varies with physical activities. Involuntary physical activities or shivering can produce heat about 3 to 5 times more than the resting level. Whereas, voluntary physical activities or exercise can produce heat about 20 to 25 times more than the resting level.

The blood levels of thermogenic hormones also generate heat by increasing metabolic rate. For example, catecholamine released by the adrenal gland in response to increased sympathetic stimulation increases the metabolic rate. Similarly, thyroid hormone released by the thyroid gland in response to prolonged or repeated exposure to a cold environment increases double the resting metabolic rate.

HEAT EXCHANGED BETWEEN THE BODY AND THE ENVIRONMENT

The exchange of heat between the body and environment occurs by four different processes. These are:

1. Radiation: It refers to a transfer of heat by infrared waves that travel through the air from warmer to colder objects. So, radiation does not require molecular contact between objects.

   As radiant heat is transmitted from a region of higher temperature to one of lower temperature, radiation is said to occur down a temperature gradient. Radiation from the sun and from objects surrounding the environment, such as walls and furniture that are warmer than the skin causes the body to gain heat. Conversely, radiation from the skin to objects in the environment that are cooler than the skin causes the body to lose at rest. Radiation is based on the principle that molecules within the body are constantly vibrating. As a result, heat is being given off in the form of electromagnetic waves.
2. Conduction: It refers to a direct transfer of heat from warmer to colder objects. In contrast to radiation, conduction requires molecular contact between objects.

As conductive heat flows from a region of higher temperature to one of lower temperature, conduction is said to occur down a temperature gradient. Therefore, temperature gradients provide the driving force for heat transfer by both radiation and conduction. For this reason, ambient temperature influences the rate at which heat can be exchanged between the body and the environment by these processes.

Conduction is a major component of heat transfer from the deep body tissues to the skin. But it becomes a minor component of heat transfer from the skin to the environment. Nonetheless, as the rate of conductive heat flow depends on both the magnitude of the temperature gradient and the thermal properties of the medium, conduction can become a significant component of heat loss in cold water because water is a better conductor of heat than air.

3. Convection: When the body temperature is higher than the surrounding air or water, heat is lost from the skin with the help of convection. The effectiveness of heat loss by conduction depends on how rapidly warmed air or water molecules are removed from the body surface. This removal of warmed molecules helps to maintain the temperature gradient. Thus, heat loss decreases when air movement (convection) is slow and increases when air movement is fast. For this reason, cycling at high speeds provide more convective cooling than does cycling at low speeds.
4. Evaporation: Heat is lost from the skin by evaporation. It occurs as a result of sweating and perspiration or insensible water loss (which refers to water removed from the body in inspired air and by diffusion through the skin).

   The sweat from our body must be changed into a gaseous water vapor at the body surface for the effective mechanism of cooling the body through evaporation. In the form of heat, energy is needed for this change and it is absorbed by the area of body surface. As the latent heat (the amount of heat needed to change 1g of water from liquid phase to the vapor phase) of water is 0.58 kcal / g, for every liter of sweat evaporated, the body dissipates approximately 580 kcal of heat energy.

   Evaporation is the major defence against overheating during exercise and it is the only mechanism by which the body can lose heat when ambient temperature exceeds skin temperature. Evaporation accounts for approximately 20 to 25% of total heat loss at rest and approximately 80% of the total heat loss during strenuous exercise.

Factors Influencing Evaporation

The driving force for evaporation of sweat is the amount by which the vapor pressure (PH_2O) at the body surface exceeds that of the surrounding air. Because vapor pressure is a function of both temperature and humidity, low ambient temperatures and relative humidity are factors that promote evaporation of sweat, whereas, high ambient temperatures and relative humidity are factors that impede evaporation of sweat. For this reason, a vigorous exercise performed in a humid environment poses a great risk of evaporated core temperature (hyperthermia) than the same exercise performed in an arid environment at the same temperature. The 'heat-stress index' provides a rating of potential risk of heat injury associated with different combinations of temperature and humidity.

Other factors that influence the rate at which sweat evaporates from the skin include the body surface area exposed to the environment (removal of clothing promotes evaporation) and the presence of convective air currents (air movement promotes evaporation).

BODY TEMPERATURE CONTROL SYSTEM

The components of the body temperature control system include:
- Thermoreceptors
- Temperature regulating system
- Effector organs.

Thermoreceptors

Body temperature is controlled by:
- Central thermoreceptors: These are situated in the hypothalamus. They detect the temperature of the body perfusing the brain.
- Peripheral thermoreceptors: These are the free nerve endings that detect the temperature of the skin. The two types of peripheral thermoreceptors are cold receptors and heat receptors. Cold receptors are more abundant and more superficially located than the heat receptors.

Temperature Regulatory Center

It is located in the hypothalamus. It receives afferent information related to core temperature from central thermoreceptors and afferent information related to environmental temperature from peripheral thermoreceptors. The cerebral cortex also receives afferent information from peripheral thermoreceptors which allows for conscious perception of skin temperature. This allows for voluntary responses to these perceptions, such as putting on or taking off clothing.

Effector Organs

The mechanisms for heat gain are coordinated by the neurons located in the posterior hypothalamus. Whereas, the mechanisms of heat loss are coordinated by the neurons located in the anterior hypothalamus. The neural output from the hypothalamus controls the activity of the effector organs of the temperature regulatory system, which include:

- Skeletal muscles
- Brown adipose tissue
- Vascular smooth muscles
- Sweat glands
- Endocrine glands.

THERMOREGULATION IN COLD STRESS

During hypothermia (low core temperature), the temperature regulatory center is stimulated by the afferent signals from the central and peripheral thermoreceptors to increase the rate of heat production by the body and to decrease the rate of heat loss to the environment. These responses cause the body to gain heat in order to restore the normal level of core temperature.

To increase heat production, the posterior hypothalamus has some responsibilities, such as:

- It stimulates the alpha and gamma motor neurons that innervate skeletal muscle that causes shivering, a rapid involuntary cycle of skeletal muscle contraction and relaxation, increasing the metabolic rate.
- It stimulates the sympathetic nerve fibers to brown adipose tissue that increases heat production.

- It initiates the release of thermogenic hormones, such as thyroxin, which too increase the metabolic rate.

  To decrease heat loss, the posterior hypothalamus has also some responsibilities such as:

- It stimulates sympathetic nerve fibers that innervate the smooth muscle of peripheral blood vessels.
- The resultant vasoconstriction decreases blood flow to the skin, decreasing the rate of heat loss of the body to the environment by radiation, conduction and convection.

THERMOREGULATION IN HEAT STRESS

During hyperthermia (high core temperature), the temperature regulatory center is stimulated by the afferent signals from central and peripheral thermoreceptors to increase the rate of heat loss to the environment. These responses cause the body to lose heat in order to restore the normal level of core temperature.

To increase the heat loss, the anterior hypothalamus serves some responsibilities:

- It stimulates the sympathetic fibers that innervate sweat glands. The resultant secretion of sweat promotes heat loss by evaporation.
- It inhibits the sympathetic fibers that innervate the smooth muscle of peripheral blood vessels.
- The resultant vasodilatation increases blood flow to the skin, which causes more heat to be lost by radiation, conduction and convection.
- Vigorous exercise, blood flow to the skin increases dramatically as evidenced by flushed skin. Because the vascular beds of different organs are arranged in parallel, it is evidenced that the blood shunted to the skin does not perfuse exercising muscles. Thus, the need to dissipate heat and prevent hyperthermia is in conflict with the need to supply fuels and oxygen to exercising muscles. The resultant competition between skin and muscle for blood flow explains why maximum exercise performance, as indicated by VO_2 max, declines in hot / humid environments.

EFFECT OF AMBIENT TEMPERATURE ON MECHANISMS OF HEAT LOSS

The temperature gradient between the skin and the environment decreases with the increase in ambient temperature, causing removal of less heat from the body by radiation, conduction and convection. Nonetheless, the total heat loss associated with a given level of submaximal exercise has been found to remain essentially constant over a wide range of ambient temperatures. This finding provides evidence that decrements in heat loss by the above mechanisms are counteracted by equal increments in heat loss by evaporation. Thus, evaporation becomes a progressively larger component of the total heat loss when ambient temperature rises.

SWEAT GLANDS

With the stimulation of sympathetic nerve fibers, the sweat glands secrete sweat. In fact, sweat is a hypotonic saline solution formed by the filtration of plasma.

There are two types of sweat glands in our body. These are:

1. The apocrine glands: They are located in the axilla and genital area. Their secretions contain a lipid substance responsible for body odor.
2. The eccrine glands: They cover most of the body. They are responsible for most of the evaporative heat loss. They consist of:
   - A deep coiled portion: It secretes an essentially odorless sweat.
   - A duct portion: It allows sweat to pass outward through the layers of the skin.

The rates of sweat production vary among individuals depending upon the genetic factors, fitness level, environmental conditions, exercise intensity, heat acclimatization and degree of hydration.

EFFECT OF SWEAT LOSS ON BODY FLUIDS

Both water and salts are lost from the body through sweating. Loss of fluids from the body is a condition called as dehydration. As we know that sweat is a hypotonic solution, the loss of water from the body is disproportionately greater than the concomitant loss of sodium and chloride. In consequences, sweat loss decreases the blood volume and increases the sodium concentration in extra-cellular fluid.

Responses to Sweat Loss

Sweat loss' activates the thirst mechanism. It is initiated by osmoreceptors in the hypothalamus that are stimulated by the higher sodium concentration in extracellular fluid. As dehydration stimulates thirst, this mechanism, by itself, is activated too late to prevent dehydration due to fluid lost by sweating during exercise. For this reason, voluntary fluid intake is recommended before and during exercise to prevent dehydration.

Sweat loss also stimulates the release of hormones that conserve water and salt, including:

Antidiuretic hormone (ADH): It is released by the posterior pituitary gland in response to a high sodium concentration in extracellular fluid. ADH increases water reabsorption by the kidney tubules. It reduces the amount of water that is excreted in urine.

Aldosterone: It is released by the adrenal cortex in response to a high potassium concentration in extracellular fluid. It increases Na^+ reabsorption by the kidney tubules and the duct portions of the sweat glands. It reduces the amount of sodium that is excreted in urine and sweat.

It is the adaptive responses to exercise in a hot environment which include:

- An expansion of blood volume.
- An earlier onset of sweating and a higher sweat rates which promotes evaporative heat loss and lower concentrations of sodium and chloride in sweat which conserves electrolytes.
- A thermoregulatory effect of an expanded blood volume is that a given increment in heat production causes a smaller rise in body temperature when more body fluid is available to absorb the added heat. A cardiovascular effect of an expanded blood volume is that a greater degree of filling of the venous circuit enhances the heart rate associated with any given cardiac output.
- The above adaptations explain why acclimatized individuals exhibit a lower heart rate and core temperature at any given level of submaximal exercise. They also explain why a reduction in blood volume due to excessive sweat loss causes a decline in maximal exercise performance.

ENVIRONMENTAL FACTORS THAT PREDISPOSE TO HYPERTHERMIA

Environmental factors that predispose to hyperthermia include:

- High ambient temperature which impairs heat loss by radiation and conduction.
- Low air movement which impairs heat loss by convection.

- High relative humidity which impairs heat loss by evaporation.
- High levels of radiant heat from the sun which increase heat gain.
- In light of the above considerations, air temperature by itself is not an accurate index of environmental heat stress.

HEAT-RELATED ILLNESS

Nearly 400 people die each year in the United States from excessive heat stress, and about half of these are men and women ages 65 years and older. If the normal signs of heat stress go unheeded—thirst, tiredness, and visual disturbances—cardiovascular compensation begins to fail. This initiates a cascade of disabling complications collectively termed heat illness. Heat cramps, heat syncope, heat exhaustion, and heat stroke constitute the major heat illnesses in order of increasing severity. When symptoms of serious heat illness occur, immediate action must include reducing heat stress and rehydrating the person until medical help arrives.

Heat-related illnesses are the complications of heat stress that include:

Heat cramps: Heat cramps refer to involuntary muscle spasms. It occurs during or after intense exercise probably due to electrolyte or body fluid imbalances.

Heat exhaustion: It is characterized by pooling of blood in dilated peripheral vessels. Its symptoms include:

- A weak rapid pulse
- Low arterial blood pressure in the upright position
- General weakness
- Dizziness
- In some cases fainting
- Heat exhaustion is comparatively more serious condition.

Heatstroke: Heatstroke is a potentially lethal condition. In this case, thermoregulation fails and body temperature rises to the point of tissue damage (more than 41.5°C). Its treatment includes:

- Alcohol rubs
- Application of ice packs
- Whole body immersion in cold water.

Heat Cramps

- Heat cramps are painful muscle spasms that occur during or after intense physical activity, usually in the specifically exercised muscles.

- Core temperature often remains within normal range.
- An imbalance in body's fluid level and electrolyte concentration produces this form of heat illness.
- Sweating causes electrolyte loss during prolonged heat exposure. Failure to replenish these minerals often leads to muscle pain and spasm, most commonly in abdomen and extremities. Prevention involves two factors:
  - (i) Providing plentiful water that contains salt.
  - (ii) Increasing daily salt intake (e.g. adding salt to foods at mealtime) several days before heat exposure.

Heat Exhaustion

It usually develops in unacclimatized persons. It occurs from ineffective circulatory adjustments compounded by depletion of extracellular fluid, principally plasma volume from excessive sweating. Blood usually pools in the dilated peripheral vessels; this drastically reduces the central blood volume necessary to maintain cardiac output. Characteristics include weak and rapid pulse, low blood pressure, headache, dizziness, and general weakness. Core temperature does not rise to dangerous levels (i.e. > 40°C). Intravenous therapy replenishes fluid effectively.

Heat Stroke

Heat stroke is the most serious and complex type of heat illness. It reflects failure of heat regulating mechanisms from an excessively high core temperature. The classic form of heat stroke – core temperature > 40.5°C, altered mental status, absence of sweating. When thermoregulation fails, sweating diminishes, the skin becomes dry and hot and body temperature rises to 41.5°C and above. This places an inordinate strain on cardiovascular function. If this condition left untreated, the disability progresses rapidly and death can occur from circulatory collapse and damage to the CNS and other organ systems. Immediate treatment includes fluid replacement, and body cooling with alcohol rubs, application of ice packs and whole body immersion in cold or even ice water.

Limit of Tolerance of Heat

The ACSM proposes the following recommendations concerning risk for heat injury with continuous exercise (e.g. endurance running and cycling) based on the WB-GT(Wet bulb-globe temperature index).

- Very high risk: Above 28°C—postpone event
- High risk: 23 to 28°C—heat-sensitive individuals (e.g. obese, low physical fitness, unacclimatized, dehydrated, history of heat injury) should not compete.
- Moderate risk: 18° to 23°C.
- Low risk: Below 18°C.

Factors that Modify Heat Tolerance

Factors that interact and affect physiologic adjustments and exercise tolerance during environmental heat stress include acclimatization, exercise training, age, gender, and body composition.

- Acclimatization.
- Relatively light exercise performed easily in cool weather becomes taxing if attempted on the first hot day of spring.
- The early stages of spring training often cause heat injury because thermoregulatory mechanisms have not adjusted to the dual challenge of exercise and environmental heat.
- Heat acclimatization refers to the physiologic adaptive changes that improve heat tolerance.

Physiologic Adjustments During Heat Acclimatization

- Acclimatization response
- Improved cutaneous blood flow
- Effective distribution of cardiac output
- Lowered threshold for start of sweating
- More effective distribution of sweat over skin surface
- Increased sweat output
- Lowered sweat's salt concentration.

Effects

- Transports metabolic heat from deep tissues to the body's shell
- Appropriate circulation to skin and muscles to meet demands of metabolism and thermoregulation; greater blood pressure stability during exercise.
- Evaporative cooling begins early in exercise.
- Optimum use of effective surface for evaporative cooling.
- Maximizes evaporative cooling.
- Dilute sweat preserves electrolytes in extracellular fluid.

Training Status

- The normal exercise-induced 'internal' heat stress from strenuous physical activity in a cool environment adjusts peripheral circulation and evaporative cooling in a manner qualitatively similar to hot ambient temperature acclimatization.

- This enables well-conditioned men and women to respond more effectively to severe heat stress than sedentary counterparts.
- Exercise training alone increases sweating response sensitivity and capacity so sweating begins at a lower core temperature. It also produces larger volumes of more dilute sweat. These beneficial responses relate to the increase in plasma volume that occurs early in endurance training.

Age

Studies that consider body size and composition, aerobic fitness level, hydration level, and degree of acclimatization show little age-related effects on thermoregulatory capacity or acclimatization to heat stress.

Gender

Women and men equally tolerate the physiological and thermal stress of exercise when matched for fitness and acclimatization levels. Gender differences occur for the following thermoregulatory mechanisms:

- Sweating: Women possess more heat-activated sweat glands per unit of skin area than men. Women begin sweating at higher skin and core temperatures; they also produce less sweat for a similar heat-exercise load, even when acclimatized comparably to men.
- Evaporative versus circulatory cooling: Despite a lower sweat output, women show heat tolerance similar to men of equal aerobic fitness at the same exercise level. Whereas women rely more on circulatory mechanisms for heat dissipation, men exhibit greater evaporative cooling. Women who sweat less to maintain thermal balance have less chance of experiencing dehydration during exercise at high ambient temperatures.

Body Fat Level

- Excess body fat negatively impacts exercise performance in hot environments. Fat's specific heat exceeds that of muscle tissue and subsequently insulates the body shell to retard heat conduction to the periphery.
- Large, overweight persons also possess a smaller body surface area-to-mass ratio for sweat evaporation compared with leaner, smaller persons.

- Excess body fat also directly adds to energy expended in weight bearing activities.
- When these effects are compounded by evaporation-retarding characteristics; the added weight of sports equipment (e.g. football uniforms and pads); intense competition; and a hot, humid environment, overweight athletes experience considerable difficult regulating their body temperature.
- Fatal heat stroke occurs 3.5 times more frequently in obese young adults than nonobese counterparts.

Acclimatization

Acclimatization refers to the body's physiologic adaptation to heat stress and increased capacity to work in the heat (Fig. 12.1). In other words, acclimatization describes the collective physiologic adaptive changes that improve heat tolerance.

- Acclimatization it is the process in a individual organism adjusting to a gradual change in its environment (such as a change in temperature, humidity, photoperiod, or pH), allowing it to maintain performance across a range of environmental conditions. Acclimatization occurs in a short period of time (days to weeks), and within the organism's lifetime (compare to adaptation).
- Process of heat acclimatization leads to improves sweating, metabolic and sympathetic responses.
- After acclimatization, there is less subjective discomfort during heat exposure, with smaller increase in pulse and respiratory rate under the same conditions of heat and activity.

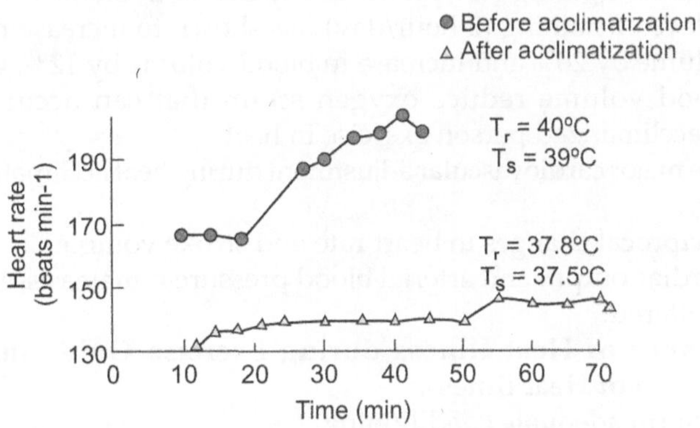

Fig. 12.1: Circulation response to heat acclimatization

- Cardiovascular stability with postural changes and activity is also greater.
- Skin and rectal temperature remains close to neutral and sweat production increases after acclimatization.
- It has been found that major acclimatization occurs during 1st week of heat response, with full acceleration thereafter. The process requires only 2-4 hours of daily heat exposure.

Physiologic adaptations/adjustments during heat acclimatization response

- Acclimatization can be facilitated by performing 5 to 10 days progressive exercise program in heat –simply sitting on bench or resting in hot environment produces little heat acclimatization.
- Exercise intensity and duration for few days of acclimatization should be reduced as low as 70% VO_2max and < 20 minute respectively.
- In addition, individual should consume as much as fluid as possible to avoid chances of heat injury.
- Exercise training conducted indoor and outdoor during winter promotes some degree of acclimatization. Exercise training produces 50 to 65% of total physiologic adjustment resulting from heat acclimatization.
- The faster onset and greater rate of sweating experienced as a result of exercise training reduces skin temperature and greatly enhances body cooling. Marked elevation in metabolic rate and increase heat production during training can cause rectal temperature to approach 40°C at end of strenuous workout which serve as stimuli for oxygenation and sweating.
- Exercise training also produces expansion in blood volume—3 days of training (2 hour/day) has shown to increase plasma volume by 20% and increase in blood volume by 12%, greater blood volume reduce oxygen strain that can occur when unacclimatized person exercise in heat.

The major cardiovascular adjustment during heat acclimatization are:

- Reciprocal changes in heart rate and stroke volume.
- Cardiac output and arterial blood pressure remains essentially unaltered.

Avoidance of Heat Illness during Exercise Guidelines for Prevention of Heat Illness:

- Perform adequate conditioning.
- Undergo acclimatization.

- *Avoid adverse conditions:* Event organizers should ensure that high intensity or endurance events should not take place in adverse conditions of heat or humidity.
- *Alter training times:* Unless trying to acclimatize, the athlete should avoid exercise at the hottest time of the day.
- Wear appropriate clothing. In hot conditions, athletes should wear loose-fitting, light-colored clothing.
- Drink appropriate amount of fluid before the event.
- The athlete should ensure that he or she is adequately hydrated in the 24 hours prior to the event.
- To minimize the uncomfortable sensations of thirst and so to optimize performance during exercise athletes can be assured that they drink only according to the dictates of their thirst. For exercise upto 1 hour in duration, plain water is appropriate.
- For exercise lasting longer than 1 hour, a dilute glucose and electrolyte solution should be used.
- *Ensure athletes and officials are well-educated*: It is important that event organizers, coaches and athletes understand the importance of adequate hydration, the danger of water intoxication, and the need to avoid excessive environmental conditions.
- *Provide proficient medical support:* A well-equipped, well-trained medical team should be present at all endurance events occurring in hot or humid conditions.

EXERCISE IN COLD

- Downhill skiing, cross-country skiing, snowboarding, backpacking, snowmobiling and ice-skating are some of the most popular outdoor activities performed in the cold.
- As the external temperature falls, various physiological thermoregulatory mechanisms are engaged to maintain the body's internal temperature.
- Although physiological mechanisms can start the adjustment processes to help keep the body warm, appropriate clothing or shelter is typically needed to meet the challenges of cold temperatures.

Three integrated factors regulate body temperature during cold exposure:

1. *Vascular adjustments:* Circulatory adjustments 'fine tune' temperature regulation. Stimulation of cutaneous cold

receptors constricts peripheral blood vessels. Vasoconstriction immediately reduces the flow of warm blood to the body's cooler surface and redirects it to the warmer core that includes cranial, thoracic, and abdominal cavities and portions of the muscle mass. Consequently, skin temperature decreases toward ambient temperature to optimize the insulatory benefits of skin, muscle and subcutaneous fat.

2. *Muscular activity:* Shivering generates metabolic heat (maximum of 3 to 5 times resting metabolism), but physical activity provides the greatest contribution in defending against cold. Exercise energy metabolism can sustain a constant core temperature when air temperatures decrease to 30°C (22°F) without the need for heavy clothing.
3. *Hormonal output:* Increased release of the 'calorigenic' hormones epinephrine and norepinephrine by the adrenal medulla partially account for increased basal heat production during cold exposure. Prolonged cold stress also increases the thyroid gland's release of thyroxine to elevate resting metabolism.

Physiological Response to Cold

The layers of tissues will alter in their temperature, as shown in the mapping of body temperature depicted by a body isotherm, at different temperatures. As temperature rises, body tissues decrease in temperature from the core to the periphery, whereas under cold conditions, body temperatures increase from the periphery to the core to preserve vital organs and the central nervous system function. This is why peripheral tissues such as skin are more sensitive to cold injury.

Physiological Response to Exercise in Cold

- Muscle functions.
  - Altered fiber recruitment → ↓ contractile force
  - Shortening velocity and power
  - Affects superficial muscles (deep muscle spared)
  - As fatigue, metabolic heat production
  - Energy reserve depletion with endurance exercise → potential for hypothermia.
- FFA metabolic responses
  - Normally, catecholamines → ↑ FFA oxidation
  - Cold → ↑ catecholamine secretion but no ↑ FFA
  - Vasoconstriction in subcutaneous fat → ↓ FFA mobilization.

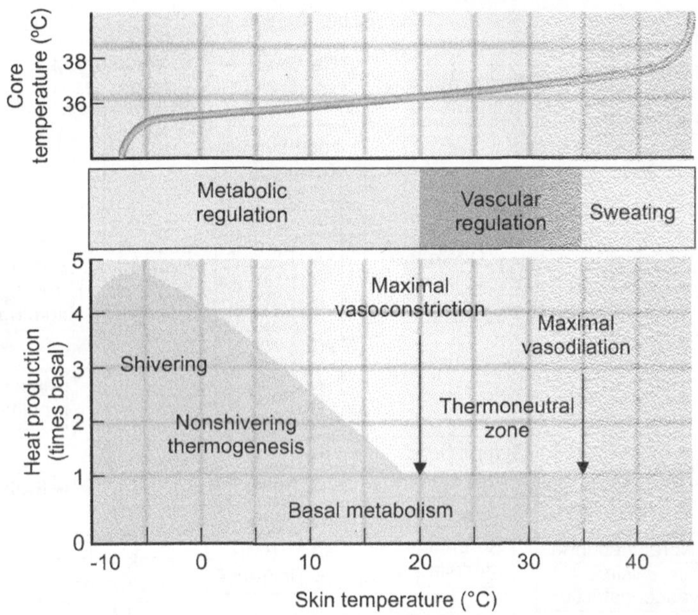

Fig. 12.2: Relationship between heat production and core and skin temperature
Source: McArdle et al., 2001

- Glucose metabolic responses
  - Blood glucose maintained well during cold exposure
  - Muscle glycogen utilization
  - Hypoglycemia suppresses shivering.

Health Risks During Exercise in The Cold

- Hypothermia
- Cardiorespiratory effects
  - Cooling primarily influences SA node leading to substantial decrease in heart rate.
  - Cold air does not damage ventilatory tissues.
  - Excessive cold affects respiratory function by decreasing respiratory rate and volume.

Body Fat, Exercise and Cold Stress

- Difference in body fat content among individuals influence physiological functions in the cold during rest and exercise.
- The additional fat increases the effective insulation in cold water when peripheral blood diverts from body's shell to the core.

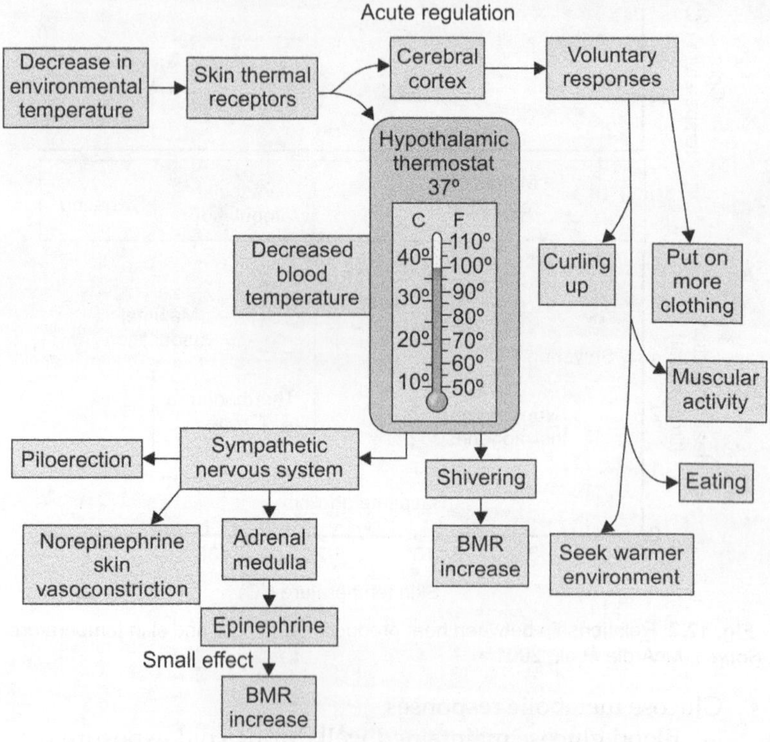

Fig. 12.3: Schematic representation of regulation of heat
Source: McArdle et al., 2001

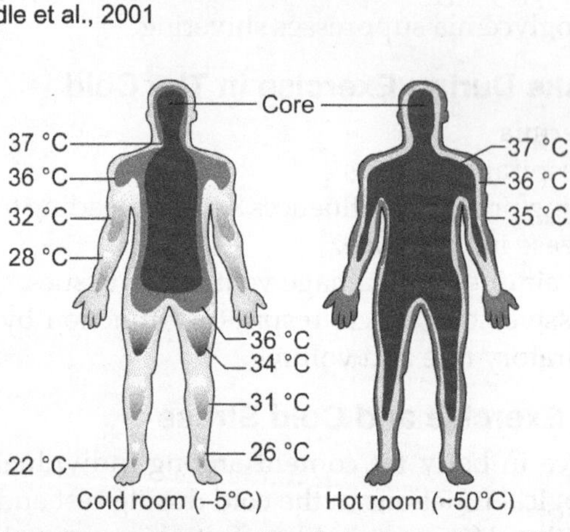

Fig. 12.4: Temperature variations in body in cold and hot room
Source: McArdle et al., 2001

- With this advantage, athletes with greater thermal insulation from fat accretion swim in cool ocean water with almost no decline in core temperature.
- For most persons water temperature between 26 and 30°C allows effective heat dissipation in sustained exercise without compromising exercise capacity from large deviations in core temperature.

Children and Cold Stress

- Cold water provides an exceptionally stressful thermoregulatory mechanism for children.
- During exercise in less stressful cold air environment, children rely on two mechanisms to compensate for their relatively large body surface area.
  - Augmented energy metabolism
  - More effective peripheral vasoconstriction in limbs.

Age

Older adults do not withstand the challenge of cold during rest and low intensity exercise as effectively as younger counterparts with similar aerobic capacities.

Age-related variations in body composition or hormonal functions may provide part of the explanation.

Gender

Women have a slight advantage over men during cold exposure because they have more subcutaneous body fat.

But their smaller muscle mass is a disadvantage in extreme cold because shivering is the major adaptation for generating body heat.

The greater the active muscle mass, greater the subsequent heat generation. Muscle also provides additional insulating layer.

Respiratory Tract During Cold Weather Exercise

Cold ambient air poses no special danger of damaging respiratory passages.

Even in extreme cold, incoming air warms to between 26 and 32°C as it reaches the bronchi, although values as low as 20°C have been observed with breathing large volumes of cold, dry air.

Warming an incoming cold air greatly increases its capacity to hold moisture. Thus, humidification of inspired cold air produces significant water and heat loss from respiratory tract, chiefly with large ventilatory volumes during exercise.

Airway moisture loss during cold weather exercise contributes to mouth dryness, a burning sensation in throat, irritation of respiratory passages and general dehydration.

Wearing a scarf or cellulose mask that covers the nose and mouth and traps the water in exhaled air (warms and moistens the next incoming breath) helps to minimize uncomfortable symptoms.

Exercise in Cold Water

Light to moderate exercise in cold water produces higher oxygen consumptions and lower body temperatures than identical exercise in warmer water.

The additional oxygen consumption directly relates to the energy cost of shivering as the body combats heat loss in colder water.

Shivering also serves an important role in recovering from hypothermia, it attenuates the typical postexercise decline in core temperature and facilitates core rewarming.

COLD ACCLIMATIZATION

- Cold habituation
  - Occurs after repeated cold exposures without significant heat loss.
  - Vasoconstriction, shivering blunted; core temperature allowed to more.
- Metabolic acclimatization
  - Occurs after repeated cold exposures with heat loss.
  - Enhanced metabolic, shivering heat production.
- Insulative acclimatization
  - When metabolism unable to maintain core temperature.
  - Enhanced skin vasoconstriction (peripheral tissue insulation).
- Precautions
  - The American Council on Exercise says it is fine to exercise in the cold as long as you take certain precautions to avoid hypothermia.

EFFECTS OF CLOTHING ON THERMOREGULATION

- Clothing insulates the body from its surroundings. It reduces radiant heat gain in a hot environment or retards conductive and convective heat loss in the cold.

- The mesh of the clothing's fibers traps air and warms it then insulate from the cold. This establishes a barrier to heat loss because cloth and air both conduct heat poorly. A thicker zone of trapped air next to the skin provides more effective insulation.
- Several layers of light clothing or garments lined with animal fur, feathers, or synthetic fabrics with numerous layers of trapped air insulate better than a single bulky layer of winter clothing.
- Wool or synthetics that insulate well and dry quickly serve this purpose.
- When clothing becomes wet, either through external moisture or condensation from sweating, it loses nearly 90% of its insulating properties. Wet clothing facilitates heat transfer from the body because water conducts heat 25 times faster than air.
- When working or exercising in cold air, the adequacy of insulation does not usually present a problem; rather, the key factor involves dissipation of metabolic heat and sweat through a thick air-clothing barrier.
- Wear layers—Insulating yourself against the wind and other elements is key, so create a layered barrier instead of a single bulk. (The advantage is you can always remove the outer layer if you get over-heated.)
- The first layer that is directly touching your skin should be a lightweight synthetic or polyester material. It will dry quickly and wick away moisture.
- The second layer should be wool or polyester fleece.
- The outermost layer—worn in the rain, snow, or wind should be lighter weight and water-repellent to help you stay dry.
- About 50% of body heat is lost from an uncovered head when the temperatures hit the freezing mark. Wearing a hat will help your body retain heat.
- Keeping hands and feet warm is key in the cold temperatures since your body will shunt blood away from extremities to keep your internal organs warm. Gloves will help to prevent skin damage and frostbite in sub-zero temperatures. To keep your feet warm, make sure your torso is properly insulated. That will drive blood back down to your lower extremities.
- Cover your face with mask or scarf when the temperature is below freezing to avoid frostbite. This can also help warm the air a bit before entering your lungs.

- Wear sturdy footwear with good traction to prevent slips and falls on snow or ice.
- Drink plenty of fluids—Staying properly hydrated is just as important during cold weather as during hot weather. Drink before, during and after your workout, even if you do not feel very thirsty, as dehydration may be more difficult to notice during cold weather exertion.
- Do not overdress—Since our bodies warm up once they get moving, we should feel cold at first. When performing higher-intensity activities, overdressing can lead to excess sweating, which will cause the body to become wet. Damp skin is an unfortunate conductor of heat loss, and will lower body temperature and increase the risk of hypothermia.
- Check the forecast—Check the air temperature and wind chill factor before exercising in the cold. The US National Safety Council says there is little risk when exercising in 20°F, even with 30 miles per hour winds, but that dangers exist when the combined temperature and windchill falls below -20°F.
- Keep in mind that wind chill can make exercising risky even if you dress warmly.

Dangers

Three primary dangers of cold weather exercise are:

1. Frostbite: Once the thermometer dips down to -6.6°C (20°F) or so, you should use extreme caution and make sure to protect your skin from exposure, as such subfreezing temperatures dramatically increase your chances of developing frostbite. Your cheeks, nose and ears are the most vulnerable, but your hands and feet are also easily affected. Early warning signs of frostbite include a stinging sensation, numbness or loss of feeling.
2. Hypothermia: Hypothermia is when core body temperature slips below 35°C (95°F) (Table 12.1). But if the heat loss is greater than body's ability to generate it, then core temperature starts to fall. As it falls, body compensates by shunting blood away from skin and towards vital organs such as heart, lungs and brain. Brain and heart are the most cold-sensitive, and as core temperature drops, the electrical activity in these organs slows.
3. Eventually, if temperature drops too low, heart and brain activity ceases altogether, and the person can die. Symptoms of hypothermia include intense shivering, slurred speech, loss of coordination and fatigue.

Table 12.1: Core temperature and associated psychological change that occur as core temperature falls, individuals respond differently at each level of core temperature

	Core temperature		
Stage	**°F**	**°C**	**Physiological changes**
Normothermia	98.6	37.0	
Mild hypothermia	95.0 93.2 91.4	35.0 34.0 33.0	Maximal shivering; increased blood pressure; amnesia; dysarthria; poor judgment; behavior change; ataxia; apathy
Moderate hypothermia	89.6 87.8 85.2 85.2	32.0 31.0 30.0 29.0	Stupor; Shivering ceases; pupils dilate Cardiac arrhythmias; decreased cardiac output Unconsciousness
Severe hypothermia	82.4 80.6 78.8 77.0 75.2 73.4 66.2 64.4 59.2 56.7	28.0 27.0 26.0 25.0 24.0 23.0 19.0 18.0 15.2 13.7	Ventricular fibrillation likely; hypoventilation Loss of reflexes and voluntary motion Acid-base disturbances; no response to pain Reduced cerebral blood flow Hypotension; bradycardia; pulmonary edema No corneal reflexes; areflex Electroencephalographic silence Asystole Lowest infant survival from accidental hypothermia Lowest adult survival from accidental hypothermia

- Treatment for mild hypothermia
  - Remove individual from cold
  - Provide dry clothing, blankets, warm beverages.
- Treatment for severe hypothermia
  - Gentle handling to avoid arrhythmias
  - Gradual rewarming
  - May require hospital facilities, medical care.
- Exercise-induced asthma: Affects upto 50% of winter-sport athletes
- Excessive airway drying
- Treated with β-agonists, steroid inhalers.

CHAPTER 13

Effects of Gender Differences on Physical Performance

Modern Olympic Games was originated in 776 BC in Greece as a tribute to the Greek god Zeus. The ancient Greek Olympics were strictly for men. Let alone competing, women were not allowed to even watch the games, considering it unethical. In fact, Olympic champions were often awarded 'a beautiful and good woman for life' (Twin, 1979). In 394 AD the games were abolished. After that it was only in 1894 in Paris, the decision to hold the first Olympiad of modern cycle was taken. The venue decided was Athens for year 1896. The man whose initiative revived the Olympic Games for athletes of all countries of the world regardless of differences of race, religion, wealth and social status, was Baron Pierre de Coubertin, also known as father of modern Olympics. But the status of women remained unaltered even then as Baron Pierre de Coubertin stated that women's sports were against the laws of nature and the most unesthetic sight human eyes could contemplate. However one woman named Melpomene did participate, against all odds, as unofficial runner in 1896 Olympics. She spent three weeks training in secret and ran 40 km from Marathon to Athens in 4.5 hours, ahead of many of the male contestants.

In 19th century, the health of woman was considered to revolve around her reproductive ability only. Any physical and psychiatric ailment was linked to the uterus. Womanly qualities of the times were beauty, chastity, modesty, obedience and inconspicuous behavior. Meek and weak wife was the status symbol of that era. Women were allowed to do only mild exercise as it was believed that overexertion would lead to hysteria. Also sweating was considered unhealthy and in addition, was socially unacceptable for women. Accepted sports for upper class women were archery, croquet, bowling, tennis, and golf (Lutter, 1994).

The period from 1920 to 1970 saw substantial progress of women in sports. Female athletes made their presence felt despite resistance to competition from physical educators, and gained worldwide attention. Helen Wills reigned as the women's tennis champion in 1920s and 30s, Gertrude Ederle swam the English channel two hours faster than anyone ever had, including men in 1926, Glenda Collett won six amateur golf championships in 1922. On the other hand, in spite of addition of five track and field events to the roster 1928, Amsterdam Olympics proved to be a disaster for female athletes as at the end of 800 m women's race several runners collapsed from heat exhaustion. Keeping this incidence in view, International Olympic Committee voted that women could not compete in races longer than 200 m leading to a 32 years ban on these races for women in Olympics.

World War II compelled the women to do the jobs requiring strength and endurance, which traditionally were considered as 'male jobs'. Even in sports women tried to fill the void created by men because of war. The confidence gained by women in tough times of war took them on the path of progress in postwar era as well. More and more women started coming forward in sports also, and then there was no turning back. The 1948 postwar Olympics in London saw 385 women participating in five sports as compared to eighteen for men making it 12.7% of the total events. In 1952, in Helsinki, 578 women from 41 countries took part and women's individual gymnastics and equestrian events were added to the roster. Physical educators began to accept and sponsor activities for high-level female athletes in the late 1960's. In 1967 Olympics in Munich, 1299 women participated making it 15% of the total participants and in 1976 Olympics in Montreal, women constituted 20.6% of the total participants. Also that year rowing and basketball were added making it 13 sports events for women to compete in. Nadia Comaneci of Romania earned the first '10' in gymnastics in the same year. In 1980 Olympics in Moscow, field hockey was added as 14th women's sport and in 1984 in Los Angeles Olympics, women were finally allowed to compete in marathon and 3,000 m. Women's cycling, synchronized swimming and rhythmic gymnastics were also added to the roster that year. In 1988 Seoul Olympics, 1,000 m cycling sprints, 10,000 m track race, heptathlon, team archery, air pistol and 50 m freestyle swimming were included. Badminton and judo for women were added in 1992 Barcelona Olympics.

Today, women are taking part in almost all kinds of sports successfully, and making their presence felt, in all sports-related professional careers. In spite of the rapid progress of females in competitive sports, it is evident that some anatomical and physiological differences are there between these two sexes which influence in their sports performances. These differences are discussed as follows.

SKELETAL DIFFERENCES

- The carpal and metacarpal bones ossify sooner in females than in males.
- X-ray assessment of the pisiform indicates that this bone is usually completely ossified in females at the age of 9 to 10 years, whereas, complete ossification in males takes place at the age of 13 years.
- Complete ossification of the metacarpal and phalanges in females occurs at the age of 16 years, whereas, in males, it occurs at the age of 19 years.
- It appears that the growth patterns of the long bones for both sexes are very similar with females' being completed 1 to 3 years sooner than males.
- This earlier ossification of bones in females does suggest a more rapid calcium metabolic rate than in their male counterparts.
- In general, a growing girl at any age has reached greater maturity than a boy of the same age in early and mid puberty.
- The rate of ossification can be changed by health, nutrition, endocrine secretions and other factors.
- The skeleton of males is more rigid, the bones are more massive and of greater density, and the long bones are somewhat longer than females.
- The joints of males are slightly larger, providing a greater articular surface than females.
- Considering the above facts, it may be stated that males have a slight advantage over females in terms of leverage and angular movement.

TRUNK, SHOULDER WIDTH AND PELVIS

- Males have wider shoulders in relation to the width of their hips, while females generally have a wider pelvis as compared to the width of their shoulders.
- The female's pelvis is more shallow than that of males (Fig. 13.1).

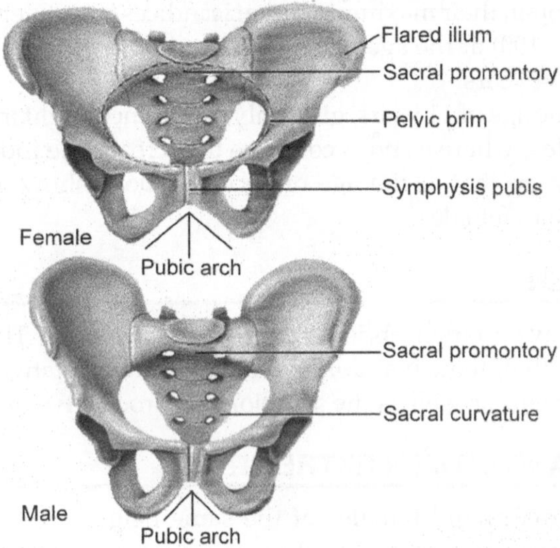

Fig. 13.1: Female and male pelvis

- Between the ages of 11 and 15 years, females have relatively wider shoulders than males. Nonetheless, after the age of 15 years, the shoulder widths of males continue to increase until at the age of 19 years, resulting somewhat larger shoulder width than that of females.
- As we know that the pelvis is comprised of two parts with each consisting of three bones, viz. (i) the ischium, (ii) pubis and, (iii) ilium. The entire pelvis is held together by several strong ligaments. In the front, the two pubis bones are separated by a cartilaginous disk. They are securely held together by other strong ligaments. During pregnancy, the action of certain female sex hormones permit the ligaments to become soft and relaxed, causing some degree of movement at the symphysis pubis and therefore expansion of pelvis.
- Women are more flexible than men.
- Women have greater range of motion in hips than men.

CHEST

- At the age of 12 and 13 years, due to the adolescent growth spurt, females generally equal or surpass males in chest circumference.
- But after the age of 13 years, males exhibit greater chest circumferences than females.

- Girls obtain their maximum thoracic indices (chest depth / chest width × 100) at the age of 11 years, and boys obtain this at the age of 14 years.
- After the age of 11 years, girls only experience slight increase in the index, whereas, boys continue to increase the index rather rapidly, so that at the age of 16 years, boys show a broader chest than females.

ABDOMEN

Females have a larger abdominal cavity than males. This is due to the fact that, female abdominal areas contain relatively larger visceral organs as well as the additional reproductive organs.

UPPER AND LOWER EXTREMITIES

- When males and females of the same height are compared, males possess generally a longer upper and forearms than females.
- Women have greater elbow flexion than men, because of shorter upper arc in olecranon process.
- Males also possess a longer length in the lower extremities than females. It is reported that men's leg length is approximately 52% of their height as compared to about 51.2% for women.
- Between the ages of 7 and 12 years, girl's leg is longer than boys. Nonetheless, after the age of 12 years, boys take over for the remainder of their lives.
- The lower legs of females are also much shorter than that of males.
- Measurements of the foot indicate that males have a greater length and breadth than that of females.

HEIGHT

- There is very little difference between males and females in height between the age of 1 and 9 years.
- After the age of about 10 years, females take the lead and with the onset of puberty, girls may outgrow their male counterparts as much as 2 inches.
- On the other hand, boys experience their growth spurt around the age of 15 years and take over the lead and never relinquish it.

- In fact, males generally continue to grow until the age of about 20 to 23 years, whereas females stop growing in height around the ages of 18 to 20 years.
- The average male is somewhere about 5 to 6 inches taller than that of the average female.

WEIGHT

- During pubertal growth, girls may weigh as much as 4 to 5 pounds more than that of males.
- Boys catch up and surpass the girls weight around the age of 15 years.
- After reaching full maturity, boys may have a total weight advantage of somewhere between 30 and 40 pounds and between 40 and 50 pounds in terms of lean body weight.

CENTER OF GRAVITY

- Center of gravity is an important aspect in physical education and sports sciences, because it determines the balance of a player. The mean center of gravity is found at a point around 56.7% of their height above ground. Whereas, the center of gravity of females is located at 56.1% of their height.
- Apparently, man's greater height, short trunk, wider shoulder and narrower pelvis account for the 0.6% difference.
- The lower center of gravity found in females is may be, due to their shorter legs and broader hips.
- Nevertheless, the lower center of gravity in females gives them an advantage over males in terms of better balance for activities like gymnastics, tumbling, etc.

ADIPOSITY

- After achieving full maturity, the average female has considerably more absolute subcutaneous fat than the average male (25% as opposed to 15% relative body fat).
- Generally females accumulate more fat in hips, thighs and in breasts than males.
- On the other hand, males possess a greater amount of fat in the upper areas of the body and in the abdominal region.

- Between the ages of 18 and 22 years, the average relative body fat of females is somewhere between 22 and 26% of the total body weight, as compared to 12 and 16% for males of same ages.
- The higher percentage of body fat of females is obviously due to their higher levels of absolute subcutaneous fat and lower levels of absolute lean body mass.
- The larger amounts of estrogen hormone, found in females, are responsible for their larger amount of body fat.
- On the other hand, the larger amounts of androgen hormones, found in males are responsible for their larger amount of lean body mass.
- This higher percentage of body fat in female athletes has some disadvantages as well as advantages too. For example, female swimmers show some 10% greater buoyancy than their male counterparts and they lose much less body heat in cold water. On the other hand, female athletes are less able to deal with hot environments than male athletes.

HEART SIZE

- Generally, male heart is larger than that of female with the exception of the 12th and 13th years.
- Mean transverse diameter of heart for men is about 12.13 cm and for women is about 10.67 cm.
- Males are physically larger and have higher percentage of lean muscle mass as compared to females.
- The heart weight to body weight ratio indicates that between the ages of 10 and 60 years, the average value for females is only 85 to 90% of the value for males, whereas after the age of 60 years, the values are similar for both sexes.

STRENGTH

- The amount and location of muscle tissue strongly effect potentials for gaining strength.
- Men appear more muscular simply because their individual muscle fibers are larger than those in women, but the quantity of fibers does not appear to differ significantly.
- Males have greater absolute strength or we can say males are approximately 30 to 40% stronger than females, as males possess

a larger muscle mass. We also know that strength potential is directly related to the physiological cross-section of the muscle.

- The greater adiposity in relation to lean muscle mass is the reason for females' lower strength to weight ratio.
- When average strength of several different muscle groups are considered as percentages of maximum strength, the average strength of both males and females is almost identical between the ages of 8 and 12 years.
- After the age of 12 years, males experience a much greater improvement in strength as compared to females, due to the influence of the male sex hormone—testosterone which brings about muscle growth.
- In fact, after the age of 12 years, both sexes continue to get somewhat stronger until they reach their twenties. Females reach their peak strength in the early to middle twenties, whereas males obtain their peak strength somewhere in the middle to late twenties.
- Following these periods, strength generally decreases with increased age.
- It is interesting to note that, below the age of 12 years, girls often surpass the boys of similar age in strength performance, such as sprints, jumps, etc.
- Nonetheless, from the age of 12 to 18 years, boys are considerably stronger in absolute strength than girls because of their tremendous muscle growth.
- Males are approximately 50 to 70% stronger in upper body strength as compared to females.
- When leg strength is expressed relative to body size, it is noted that the two sexes are the same.
- When leg strength is calculated in terms of relative to lean body weight, males are approximately 5.8% weaker than females.
- The quality of muscle in terms of its ability to contract and exert force is identical in both sexes. The similarities in leg strength between the sexes are may be, due to the similarities in use, such as walking, riding cycles, climbing stairs, etc.
- On the other hand, females traditionally do not use their upper body to the same degree as males in masculine activities such as throwing, lifting, rope climbing, etc. resulting less strength in upper body.

- Men appear to have larger slow and fast twitch fibers than women.
- Men appear to demonstrate larger absolute increases in strength and degree of muscle hypertrophy than women when both undergo identical weight training regimens.
- Women and men make same relative gain in muscular hypertrophy after a resistance training program.
- Women showed lesser relative strength increase than men because muscle cross-sectional area is directly related to ability to produce force.
- Muscle cross-sectional area is two times greater in males than females in body building.
- Women have lower proportion of their total lean body mass in their upper body so this may warrant additional upper strength training.
- An average women responds to weight training with slight increase in muscle girth and decrease in intramuscular and subcutaneous fat stores, little change in limb circumference.
- Women gain relative strength at the same rate as men when performing identical resistance training program because women begin weight training regimes at lower resistance than men.

BLOOD VOLUME AND HEMOGLOBIN

- Trained and untrained males have a greater blood volume and total hemoglobin content than trained and untrained females.
- In fact, on an average, males have about 15% more hemoglobin per 100 mL of blood than females.
- Males have an average resting red blood cell count of about 5,000,000 per cubic mm as compared with 4,500,000 per cubic mm in females.
- These factors suggest that males have greater oxygen-carrying capacity than females.

BLOOD PRESSURE

- Before menopause, women have about 5 to 10 mm Hg lower systolic and diastolic blood pressures than men of the same ages.
- After menopause, blood pressure of females tends to increase slightly over that of males.

HEART RATE

- Males possess a larger heart than females, may be due to their more muscular tissue which requires better circulation than the contrasting proportion of adipose tissue in females.
- Males have a greater heart volume than females.
- Women have resting heart rate 5 to 10 beats faster than men because of the heart size difference.
- Albeit, the maximum heart rate in both men and women at a given age is very similar, during submaximal work, the heart rate of women has been found to be considerably higher. The fact indicates that, for any given exercise, females work at a higher percentage of their maximal heart rate per oxygen uptake rate than males.

STROKE VOLUME AND CARDIAC OUTPUT

- At rest, in the supine position, the stroke volume of an adult untrained man is around 70 to 100 mL per beat depending upon the body size.
- Women have usually around 25% lower stroke volume than men because of their smaller heart size.
- During submaximal work also, stroke volume of women is lower than men.
- In standing position, stroke volume is about 30% smaller in both the sexes.
- Research findings suggest that at submaximal workload, cardiac output per liter of oxygen uptake is higher in women than in men (around 1.5 L higher).
- During exercise, both maximal cardiac output and maximal stroke volume is lower in females than males.
- Maximal arteriovenous oxygen difference is also lower in females than males during exercise.
- The hemoglobin concentration in women is lower than men.
- The arterial oxygen content is also lower in women than men.

OXYGEN PULSE

- It is generally defined as the amount of oxygen taken out of blood per heartbeat. Between the ages of 12 to 15 years, the oxygen pulse values are same for both sexes.

- From the ages of 15 to 25 years, male's value continues to improve until they are almost double the value of females.
- Female's value of oxygen pulse remains relatively the same with very little increase after the age of 15 years.

VITAL CAPACITY

- Vital capacity is defined as the maximal volume of air which a person can expel from his/her lungs by a forcible expiration after the deepest possible inspiration. It is related to age, body weight, height and skin surface area.
- For normal, healthy females, lung capacity is approximately 10% smaller than that of males of similar age and size. This difference may be due to the lower metabolic rate of females which demands less oxygen.
- Some authorities feel that the difference is due to a higher per minute respiratory rate of females than most males.
- The other authorities have suggested that the difference may be due to males' more developed respiratory musculature.
- In fact, on the average, men have a tendency to breathe somewhat slower and deeper with their abdominal and diaphragm muscles than women. At the same time, women tend to breathe faster and higher up in their chest region using the intercostals muscles. Studies show that diaphragmatic breathing can be increased in females with adequate training program.
- The average vital capacity in normal untrained adult males is around 4 L, and for the untrained females, around 3.5 L. Some authorities have found the average vital capacity of between 4.5 and 6.0 L for well-trained college females and males respectively.

MAXIMAL VOLUNTARY VENTILATION

- Maximal voluntary ventilation or maximal breathing capacity is defined as the maximal volume of air that can be moved in and out of the lungs per unit time.
- For healthy, untrained men of 25 years of age, the mean value is about 140 L/min. For women, the normal value ranges somewhat between 70 and 120 L.
- It is well-documented that maximal voluntary ventilation can be increased by training.

- Research findings report the values as high as between 200 and 250 L/min in well-trained athletes.

MAXIMUM OXYGEN UPTAKE

- Maximum oxygen uptake is defined as the greatest oxygen uptake attained by an individual while breathing air sea level, during the performance of physical work.
- It is considered as the best single measure of an individual's cardiorespiratory capacity.
- Upto the ages of between 10 and 15 years, there is very little difference in maximum oxygen uptake between girls and boys.
- Nevertheless, in adults, the capacity of women is considerably below that of men. These differences are probably due to females' lower hemoglobin count and lower maximal cardiac output than men. Sedentary lifestyle of females that society imposes on them, once they reach menarche, may be another reason for this difference.
- As there is very little difference in maximum oxygen uptake up to the ages of between 10 and 15 years, it can be stated that both sexes are very similar in hemoglobin levels and maximal cardiac output upto puberty.
- Both sexes peak their maximum oxygen uptake at around the ages of 18 to 20 years, followed by a progressive decline throughout the remaining years.

BASAL METABOLIC RATE

- Basal metabolic rate is defined as the minimum amount of energy required for each square meter of body surface area during a state of complete rest.
- It is generally well-recognized that women oxidize their food approximately 5 to 10% slower than men. Therefore, their basal metabolic rate is about 5 to 10% lower than men at all ages.
- The difference begins to increase slightly at puberty and continues until around the age of 20 years. After that time, a gradual decline commences.
- Between the ages of 20 and 40 years, women usually average about 35 kcal/m^2 of body surface area per hour in caloric expenditure, which over a period of 24 hours, will result in basal rates ranging from 1200 to 1400 kcal.

- On the other hand, between the same ages and comparable body structure, men show values around 38 kcal/m^2 of body surface area and basal rates for a 24 hour period of somewhere around 1668 kcal.
- The overall smaller size of females and greater proportion of adipose tissue to their lean body mass are probably responsible for this difference.

HEAT ADAPTATION

- In earlier chapter, it has been discussed that the temperature regulating mechanism of both men and women are somewhat different. For example, estrogen, the female sex hormone, inhibits sweating to some degree. As a result, females possess about 2° to 3° F higher sweating threshold than men. This means that females do not commence sweating until the environmental temperature is 2° to 3° F above the males' sweating threshold. As a result, the sum of sweating of females at higher temperatures will be less than that of the males.
- Another difference between the sexes in terms of heat adaptation is that the temperature gradient from core to skin appears to be smaller for females.
- Females have about 10% more adipose tissue than males which serves as good heat insulation.
- These combined findings indicate that, in a hot climate, the physiological cost of maintaining heat balance is not only greater for females, but it apparently hinders their physical performance more significantly than it does for males.
- Because females have approximately 10% more adipose tissue than males, they are somewhat better able to cope with cold conditions such as channel swimming, snow skiing, etc. than males.

CHAPTER 14

Manipulation of Body Composition Status in Athletes

HUMAN BODY COMPOSITION

The human body consists of several levels of structural organization. They are associated with one another in various ways. Considering the increasing stages of complexity, five levels of body composition can be envisioned (Wang et al. 1992). Each level is distinct and inclusive and at each level, the sum of the components equals the body mass (Fig. 14.1).

Atomic Level

The fundamental components of the body are included in the atomic level. Though more than 50 different atoms are found in the body, the vast majority located in various tissues and organs are oxygen, carbon, hydrogen, nitrogen, calcium, and phosphorus, which constitute about 98% of body mass. The prime element, oxygen, represents more than 60% of body weight. Rest of the remaining 44 elements, of which the predominant are potassium, sulfur, sodium, chloride, and magnesium, only make up 1% of body mass.

Molecular Level

Major eleven elements in the body are incorporated into compounds that represent the molecular level of body composition. These essential molecules include water, lipid or fat, protein, mineral and glycogen. The molecular level is very much important because it provides the conceptual basis for subsequent levels of organization that follow, and a link with biochemistry and energy metabolism which relate body structure and functions. The molecular level of body composition is given much emphasize, because its components are most frequently measured in studies of physical activity. The classical cadaver analysis reveals five major

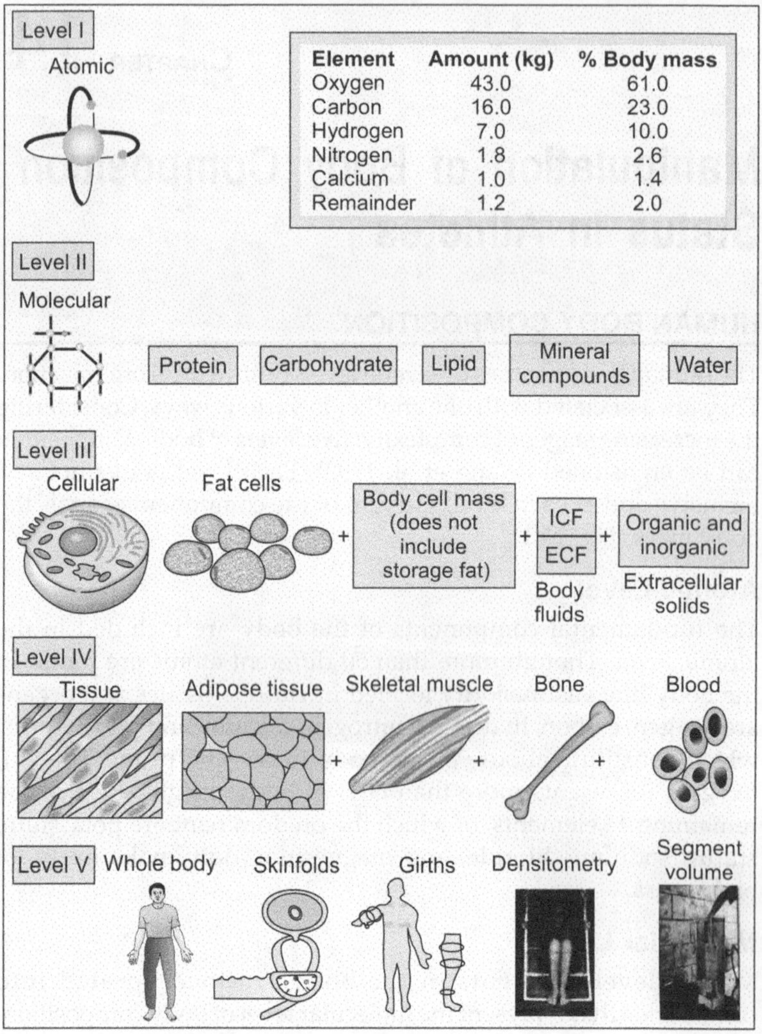

Fig. 14.1: Five levels of body composition

components of the body viz. (i) fat, (ii) water, (iii) protein, (iv) bone minerals, and (v) nonbone or soft tissue minerals. Although another component glycogen, may be incorporated and, its limited amount precludes its determination.

This molecular model can be further divided into functional components viz. fat and fat-free mass. The fat-free mass, which represents the metabolically active tissue, is distinct from fat mass because of chemical and physical characteristics. Fat has a lower density (0.900 vs. 1.100 g/cc) than the fat-free mass and does not contain water or potassium. The individual components of the fat-free body (water, bone mineral and cell mass) can be determined with appropriate methods.

Cellular Level

The cellular level of body composition accumulates the components of the molecular level into the cells that comprise the human body. Four groups of cells can be characterized as muscle, nerve, connective and epithelial cells. The connective cells constitute a multifunctional group which includes adipocytes, osteocytes and blood cells. In this compositional model there are also extracellular components, fluids and solids. The extracellular fluid is the non-metabolizing fluid which surrounds all cells. It contains about 95% water and is distributed between the plasma and the interstitial fluid which are estimated to be about 5% and 20% of body mass, respectively. The extracellular solids also are nonmetabolizing components of the body. These include organic compounds, such as collagenous, reticular and elastic fibers, and inorganic compounds, mainly dry bone matrix or calcium hydroxyapatite, magnesium, sodium, citrate, and bicarbonate.

Tissue-System Level

The combination of cells and extracellular components is responsible to form the tissue and systems levels of body composition. The tissues are commonly categorized as muscular, nervous, connective, and epithelial. In fact, bone, muscle, and adipose tissue constitute more than 75% of body mass. The body contains 11 systems, such as digestive, respiratory, circulatory, integumentary, nervous, muscular, endocrine, lymphatic, skeletal, reproductive and excretory, and the components of different systems, too, possess multiple organs that share an integrated function.

Whole-body Level

The combination of the components of these four above-mentioned levels culminates in the whole-body or the fifth level of body composition. The human body is characterized by size (stature and mass), shape, and its various dimensions (limb and trunk lengths and their circumferences). Importantly, biological and genetic processes have immense influence on all these levels of body composition. Therefore, functional adaptations associated with physical activity have profound impact in structural changes or alterations in the components at all levels of body composition.

ELEMENTARY COMPOSITION OF HUMAN BODY

Elementary components of our body are as follow:

- Oxygen 65%
- Carbon 8%
- Hydrogen 10%
- Nitrogen 3%
- Calcium 1.25%
- Phosphorus 1.00%
- Potassium 0.35%
- Sulfur 0.25%
- Chlorine 0.15%
- Magnesium 0.05%
- Iron 0.004%
- Iodine 0.00004%.

Apart from these, copper, zinc, fluorine, silicon, cobalt, molybdenum, etc. are also found in human body.

BODY COMPOSITION MODELS

Direct measurement of body composition in living human is not feasible, so various models for indirect estimation of the constituents of the body have been developed.

The two component chemical model has been the primary one, used in the study of the relationship between body composition and physical performance. This model divides the body into fat mass (FM) and fat-free mass (FFM). Fat is a molecular level component, which are cellular and tissue system components of body composition. The terms fat and lipid are often confused and inappropriately interchange (Heymsfield and Wang, 1993). Fat refers to the family of chemical compounds called triglycerides, whereas lipid is the more general term that includes triglycerides and many other compounds, e.g. glycerophosphatides and sphingolipids (Gurr and Harwood, 1991). In the two component chemical model, the fat component has included all lipids and all other body constituents are included in the fat-free mass. In more complex three or four component chemical models, the FFM is subdivided into its major constituents viz. water, mineral and protein (Boileau and Lohman, 1977).

The evaluation of body composition allows quantification of the major structural components of the body muscles, bone and fat. Although height-weight tables are still widely used to assess the extent of 'over weightness' based on age and 'frame size' such tables do not provide reliable information with regard to relative composition or quality of individual body weight (McArdle et al. 2001).The studies on body composition also assess quantitatively the amount or proportions of major fatty tissue, muscular tissue and skeletal tissue.

The total amount of body fat exists in two depots or storage sites. The first depot termed essential fat, is the fat stored in the marrow of bones as well as in the heart, lungs, liver, spleen, kidneys, intestine, muscles and lipid-rich tissues throughout the central nervous system. This fat is required for normal physiologic functioning. In females, essential fat also includes sex specific fat or sex characteristic fat.

The storage fat is that which comprises the adipose tissue or adipocytes. The number of adipocytes generally becomes fixed around 9 to 12 months after birth of the child. This nutritional reserve includes fatty tissues that protect the various internal organs from trauma and the larger subcutaneous fat volume deposited beneath the skin surface. Although the proportional distribution of storage fat in males and females is similar (12% in males, 15% in females), the total percentage of essential fat in females, which includes the sex specific fat, is 4 times higher than in males. Women at some stage in their lives may nourish a fetus and then baby from their own reserve. They have to stock energy in the form of fat for childbearing and other hormone-related functions.

We have two types of adipose tissue in our body. These are: (i) white and (ii) brown. In well-nourished adults, white adipose tissue makes up 20 to 25% of body weight. It is found between muscle fibers, supporting the kidneys and the eyes, and under the skin where it acts as thermal insulator. Brown adipose tissue is present in relatively small quantities and is situated mainly between the scapular, in the nape of the neck and in the walls of the large blood vessels of the trunk. Brown adipose tissue has a more extensive capillary network than white adipose tissue. When it is metabolized, it produces considerably more heat and less energy, contributing to the maintenance of body temperature.

In the proposed theoretical model of body fat distributed for Behnke's (1969) reference female. For woman, as part of the 5 to 9% sex specific reserve storage fat, the breasts contribute approximately 4.4% of the total mass of body fat, or no more than 12.5% to the quantity of sex specific fat (McArdle et al. 2001).There are other substantial sex specific depots in the females such as pelvic, buttock and thigh regions that contribute quantitatively to female body fat stores (Rubeffe Scrive, 1985).

The lean body mass contains a small percentage of essential fat stores (Perhaps as much as 3%) chiefly within the central nervous system, marrow of bones, and internal organs. In contrast, use of the term 'fat-free mass' refers to the body mass devoid of all extractable fat. Behnke (1969) points out that the fat-free mass is an *in vitro* entity, and is the appropriate term with regard to carcass analysis. He once again, views the lean body mass, on the other hand, is an *in vivo* entity that remains relatively constant throughout the active adult lifespan with respect to water, organic matter and minerals. In normally hydrated, healthy adults, the only difference between the fat-free mass and lean body mass is the 'essential' lipid-rich stores in bone marrow, brain, spinal cord and internal organs.

Body composition analysis is important in many fields like that of human biology, human genetics, physical anthropology, sports medicine, physiotherapy, occupational health, geriatrics, preventive medicine, physical education, home sciences, etc. Measurements of body composition provide sensitive indices of body fatness and therefore a mean of describing relatively subtle changes in energy balance, which may have the potential influence performance or in the longer form of healthy life, excessive amount of body fat is associated with many diseases and disabilities. Researches indicate that over-fat individuals are often hypertensive and have elevated serum-lipid level. Mechanical disabilities like flat feet, osteoarthritis of knee, hip, lumbar spine, abdominal hernias, diaphragmatic hernias, varicose veins, respiratory infections are associated with obesity. The health risks of obesity also include autonomic and ventricular dysfunction, adult onset diabetes mellitus, renal disease, problems in administering anesthetics during surgery, several types of cancer, menstrual irregularities and enormous psychological burden.

BEHNKE'S REFERENCE MAN AND REFERENCE WOMAN

Different body composition components for the reference man and reference woman are shown in Figures 14.2 and 14.3 respectively. The figures represent total body mass into lean body mass, muscle, and bone with total body fat categorized into storage and essential fat on the basis of data from laboratory studies of tissue composition and structure, Behnke (1969) expressed the theoretical model for the body composition of the reference man (Fig. 14.2) and reference woman (Fig. 14.3).

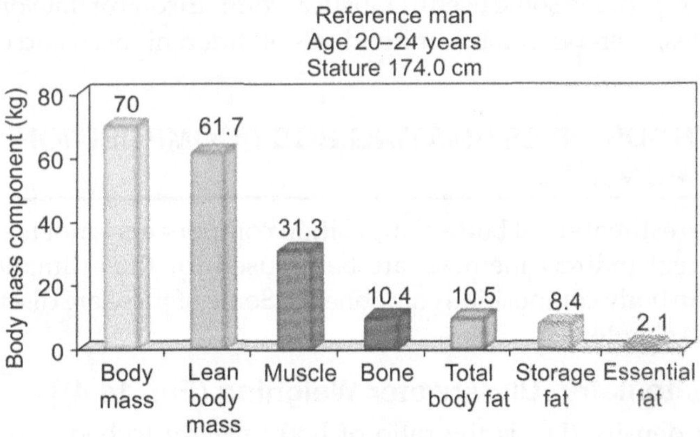

Fig. 14.2: Behnke's reference men

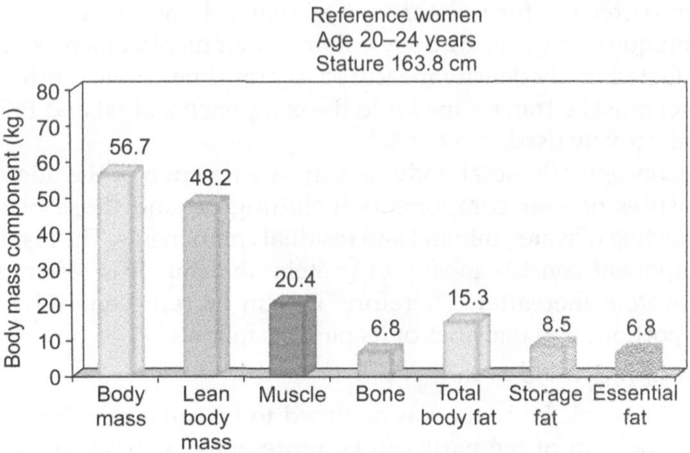

Fig. 14.3: Behnke's reference women

Comparing Figures 14.2 and 14.3, it is clear that the reference man is taller and heavier, having more skeletal weight, larger muscle mass and lower body fat content than the reference woman. These differences are also evident when muscle, fat and bone are considered as a percentage of body mass. Number of factors is responsible for the differences of the percentage of these body composition components between the two sexes. Differences in lifestyle, hormonal, structural, physiological, etc. are some of those. The concept of reference standards does not mean that every individual will achieve it by hook or by crook. In fact these reference models provide some useful statistical comparisons of data on elite athletes, exercise trainees, individuals of different racial and ethnic groups.

METHODS OF ESTIMATING BODY COMPOSITION COMPONENTS

In vivo estimation of body composition components is not feasible. Different indirect methods are being used for the estimation of human body composition components. Some of these are discussed in this chapter.

Densitometry [Underwater Weighing (Fig. 14.4)]

Body density (D_B) is the ratio of body weight to body volume. Total body volume is normally measured by hydrostatic weighing with correction for pulmonary residual volume. A more recent technique for measuring body volume by air displacement is being evaluated. Body density measured as grams per cubic centimeter (g/cc) must be transformed into the components of fat and FFB to be effectively used.

Conceptually, total body density is a function of the additive densities of four components including fat and those of FFB consisting of water, mineral and residual components. The residual component consists mostly of protein and thus it is referred to as protein thereafter. Therefore, D_B can be represented by the proportions and densities of its parts as follows:

$$D_B = 1 / (f/d_f + w/d_w + m/d_m + p/d_p) \quad (1)$$

The whole body mass is assumed to be equal to unity (one); thus the sum of the parts can be represented as fractions of the whole accordingly $1 = f + w + m + p$. The lower case letters (f, w,

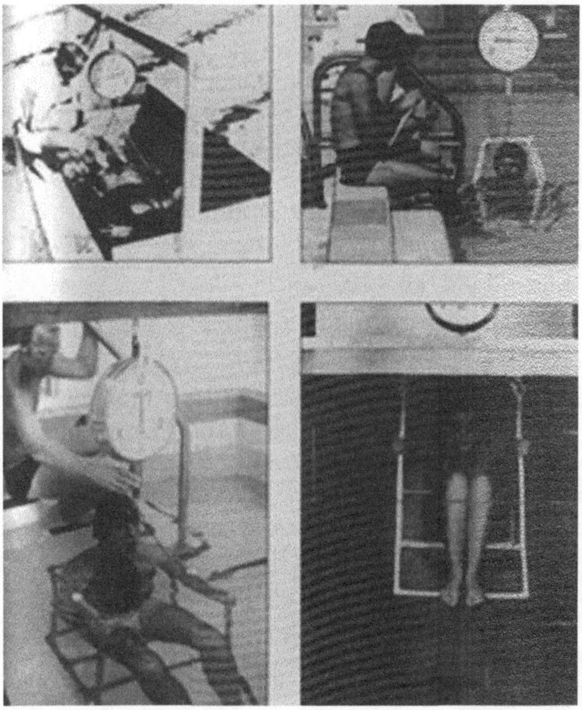

Fig. 14.4: Underwater weighing

m, p) represent the fractions of fat, water, mineral, and protein respectively and lower case letter d with its subscribes indicates the densities of the individual components. This formulation is the basic of several densitometric models.

Among the densitometric body – composition paradigms the two component model, consisting of fat and FFB, is the most commonly used. Several equations have been developed based on both theoretic and empiric assumptions associated with the two component model. To estimate % fat from densitometry by using the two-component model, assumptions are made about the densities of both components based on adult cadaver date. Because fat is a solitary component, it is reasonable to assume that the density of fat, 0.900 g/cc, is somewhat constant with regard to proportions of its respective components is less tenable, particularly during growth and aging. Moreover there is variability in the FFB component among racial groups, which is of considerable importance in the athletic population. Most of the body composition literature on the athletes is based on the Siri (1961) equation, which was derived through the two component model by assuming the constants for the density of fat (D_f) of 0.900 g/cc and the density of FFB (D_{FFB}) of 1.100 g/cc by using the following general equation:

$$\% \text{ fat} = 1/D_B [(D_f \times D_{FFB}) / D_{FFB} - D_f)] - [D_f / (D_{FFB} - D_f)] \times 100 \quad (2)$$

By using these constants for D_f and D_{FFB} in eq. (2), the Siri's equation can be formulated as follows:

$$\% \text{ fat} = (4.95 / D_B - 4.50) \times 100 \quad (3)$$

Fat-free body mass is calculated as:

$$\text{FFB} = \text{Body weight (BW)} - (\%\text{fat}/100) \times \text{BW} \quad (4)$$

To use the most appropriate equation for estimating % fat from D_B, the D_{FFB} representative of the group being assessed must be known to compute accurate body composition estimates. Unfortunately, information on the D_{FFB} for age and racial groups is extremely sparse and as yet no studies have defined the variability in D_{FFB} among athletic groups. Recent work in this regard has focused on measuring the D_{FFB} during various stages of growth and development.

There appears to be consensus that the D_{FFB} changes at various stages of the growth process and that specific equations are needed to adjust for changes in the D_{FFB} more accurately to estimate fat and FFB of children and adolescents. Several review articles have summarized the available data pertaining to variability in D_{FFB} during growth and development (Boileau and Lohman, 1997). The following equations have been proposed to account for the apparent growth-related changes in the D_{FFB} and are recommended for the adolescent athletes to estimate %fat from body density:

Boys aged 13 to 15 years: $\%\text{fat} = (5.075 / D_B - 4.639) \times 100$ (5)

Girls aged 13 to 15 years: $\%\text{fat} = (5.119/ D_B - 4.688) \times 100$ (6)

Boys aged 15 to 17 years: $\%\text{fat} = (5.033/D_B - 4.592) \times 100$ (7)

Girls aged 15 to 17 years: $\%\text{fat} = (5.075/D_B - 4.639) \times 100$ (8)

The importance of using the appropriate equations for estimating %fat from D_B is two fold. The estimation of target body weight at a recommended %fat depends on an accurate estimation of the FFB. Moreover, the D_B method is the primary method for the calibration and validation of other more clinically useful methods including anthropometry, biolectric impendence and infrared interactance. Thus development of equations for these clinical methods should use the most relevant equation for estimating body composition from D_B for the cohort being assessed.

Clinical Methods for Assessing Body Composition

Whereas densitometry generally offers better accuracy and precision, its application is restricted to a laboratory setting, is limited in availability and depends on expensive technology. Additionally, it requires considerable subject cooperation and/or a lengthy measurement process. Methods that provide rapid, safe, inexpensive, accurate and precise body-composition measurements can be useful for testing athletes in the clinical and field testing setting.

Body Mass Index (BMI)

Although BMI cannot be technically classified as a body-composition measurement method, it has received widespread use with adults for clinical and epidemiologic assessments. The BMI requires measurement only of height (H) and body weight. It is defined as BW / H^2 and expressed as kg/m^2. The development of BMI norms from large data bases permits the classification of individuals into categories of underweight, normal weight, overweight and obese. Use of the BMI has been criticized on grounds that the numerator, BW is influenced not only by fat but also by the FFB. Indeed it can be shown that most heavy weight athletes (e.g. weight lifters, football linemen, and shot putters) are classified as overweight, if not as obese, by their index when in fact their %fat estimates based on body-density measurements are normal for their sport peer group. The same observations have been made for female basketball and volleyball players. Because most athletes have a higher FFB weight, largely because of increased muscle mass, the BMI is of little value in evaluating the athlete and thus is not recommended.

Skinfold Method (Fig. 14.5)

To predict body fatness, measurement of subcutaneous fat is done by skinfold method with reasonable accuracy in laboratory as well as in field. The rationale for using skinfold method comes from interrelationship among three factors viz. (i) subcutaneous fat, (ii) internal fat, and (iii) whole-body density. Harpenden skinfold caliper is widely used for the measurement of skinfold thickness. Lange and common plastic calipers are also used for this purpose.

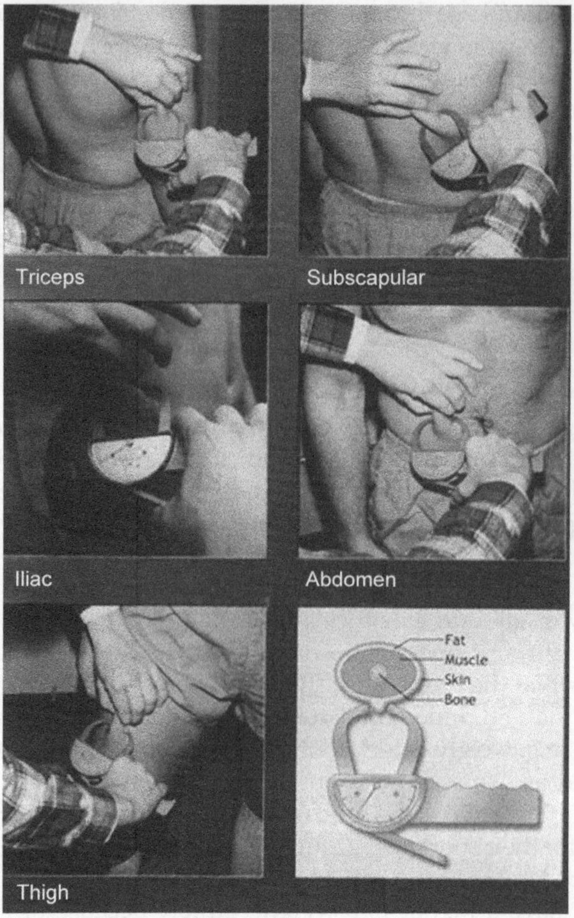

Fig. 14.5: Skinfold measurements

Skinfold measurement provides considerably meaningful and consistent information about subcutaneous fat and its distribution. Generally two ways are recommended to use skinfolds.

The first one is the sums of the skinfold scores which indicate relative fatness among individuals. For this purpose measure triceps, biceps, subscapular and suprailiac skinfolds. Then add up the four reading. The percent body fat of males and females can be determined following Tables 14.1 and 14.2 respectively.

For example, assume a 36-year-old man is being measured, and the sum of the four skinfold reading is 50 mm to the 30 to 39 age columns on. Table 14.1 his percent body fat could be estimated as 23.0% or if a 20-year-old woman were being measured, and the sum of the four skinfold measurements were 28 mm. The 16 to 29 years age column on Table 14.2 would show her percent body fat to be 18.6%.

Note that there is not a single line for every millimeter or column for every age group on the tables. To do this would make the tables too large and unwieldy. Therefore, if greater accuracy is desired, it is necessary to interpolate. For example, a woman in the 16 to 29 years of age group could have a sum of 29 mm for the four skinfolds. This is halfway between 28 and 30 on the table. The %body fat for 28 mm is 18.6% and that for 30 is 19.5%. Interpolating halfway between would give approximately 19.0%.

When interpolating for age, note that the tables are most accurate for someone whose age is in the middle of each group, so that the 30 to 39 years age group will be most accurate for someone about 34-year-old. For a person 29 or 30 years, the most accurate result will be obtained by interpolating between the two age groups. For example, a 29-year-old woman with a sum of 40 mm would obtain 16.3% body fat from the 16 to 29 column (Table 14.1), and 20.3% from the 30 to 39 column (Table 14.1). Interpolating halfway between would give a more accurate value of 18.3%.

The second use of the skinfolds incorporates population specific mathematical equation for the prediction of body density or percentage body fat. For the subjects similar in age, gender, fatness, training status, sports events and race, the equations have been proved to be accurate enough. Fulfilling all these criteria, predicted body fat for an individual usually ranges between 3 and 5% body fat units.

Considering triceps skinfold (TS) and subscapular skinfold (SS) in young women and men, the body fat can be predicted with the formula:

For young women (ages 17-26 years)

% Body fat = 0.55 TS + 0.31 SS + 6.13

For young men (ages 17-26 years)

% Body fat = 0.43 TS + 0.58 SS + 1.47

For both the equations, TS is triceps skinfold and SS is subscapular skinfold (mm). Among the young adults, the subcutaneous body fat comprises about half of the body's total fat. Proportionately more fat deposits internally than subcutaneously with the advancement of age. Therefore, the same skinfold score projects comparatively greater total percentage of body fat as a person gets older. So, in older men and women, age adjusted generalized equations should be used to predict body fat from skinfold.

Applying the surface area formula, the validity of body fat estimation in diverse populations may be improved upto a considerable level. Albeit, the method has limitations of its own. The basic equation is % fat = E skinfold ÷ 3 F × K (SF)

Where, E skinfolds is the sum of scores of two or more skinfolds, depending on availability; $3F = \sqrt{mass / stature}$ (with body mass in kg and stature is in cm) and K = (SF) is skinfolds/3F × %fat.

Table 14.1: Percent body fat of males from sum of biceps, triceps, subscapular and suprailiac skinfolds

Sum of 4 skinfolds	Age groups			
	16–29	30–39	40–49	50+
16	6.7	9.3	9.5	9.7
18	7.9	10.8	10.9	11.0
20	8.1	12.0	12.2	12.5
22	9.2	13.0	13.5	13.9
24	10.2	13.9	14.6	15.1
26	11.2	14.7	15.7	16.3
28	12.1	15.5	16.7	17.4
30	12.9	16.2	17.6	18.5
35	14.7	17.8	19.7	20.8
40	16.3	19.2	21.5	22.8
45	17.7	20.4	23.1	24.7
50	19.0	21.5	24.6	26.3
55	20.2	22.5	25.9	27.8
60	21.2	23.5	27.1	29.1
65	22.2	24.3	28.2	30.4
70	23.2	25.1	29.3	31.5
75	24.0	25.9	30.2	32.6
80	24.8	26.6	31.2	33.7
85	25.6	27.6	32.1	34.6

Contd...

Contd...

Sum of 4 skinfolds	Age groups			
	16–29	30–39	40–49	50+
90	26.3	28.3	32.9	35.5
95	27.0	29.0	33.8	36.5
100	27.6	29.7	34.5	37.3
110	28.8	30.9	35.8	38.8
120	29.9	32.0	37.1	40.2
130	31.0	33.0	38.2	41.5
140	31.9	34.0	39.4	42.8
150	32.8	34.8	40.4	43.9
160	33.6	35.7	41.4	45.0
170	34.4	36.5	42.3	46.0
180	35.2	37.2	43.1	47.0
190	35.9	37.9	43.9	47.9
200	36.5	38.6	44.7	48.8

Table 14.2: Percent body fat of females from sum of biceps, triceps, subscapular and suprailiac skinfolds

Sum of 4 skinfolds (mm)	Age groups			
	16–29	30–39	40–49	50+
14	9.4	12.7	15.6	17.0
16	11.2	14.3	17.2	18.6
18	12.7	15.7	18.5	20.1
20	14.1	17.0	19.8	21.4
22	15.4	18.1	20.9	22.6
24	16.5	19.2	22.0	23.7
26	17.6	20.1	22.9	24.8
28	18.6	21.1	33.8	25.7
30	19.5	21.9	24.6	26.6
35	21.6	23.8	27.2	28.6
40	23.4	25.5	28.1	30.3
45	25.0	27.0	29.6	31.9
50	26.5	28.3	30.9	33.2
55	27.8	29.5	32.1	34.6

Contd...

Contd...

Sum of 4 skinfolds (mm)	Age groups			
	16–29	30–39	40–49	50+
60	29.1	30.6	33.2	35.7
65	30.2	31.6	34.2	36.7
70	31.2	32.6	35.1	37.7
75	32.2	33.5	38.7	38.8
80	33.1	34.3	36.8	39.5
85	34.0	35.2	38.4	40.4
90	34.8	36.0	39.1	41.1
95	35.6	36.7	39.9	41.9
100	36.3	38.4	40.6	42.6
110	37.7	38.7	41.8	43.9
120	39.0	39.9	43.0	45.1
130	40.2	41.1	44.1	46.2
140	41.3	42.1	45.1	47.3
150	42.3	43.1	46.0	48.2
160	43.2	44.0	46.9	49.1
170	44.6	45.1	47.8	50.0
180	45.0	45.6	48.5	50.8
190	45.8	46.4	49.3	51.6
200	46.6	47.1	50.0	52.3

Measurements of Girths

Apply a linen or plastic measuring tape (not a metal tape) lightly to the skin surface so that the tape remains fixed but not tight. This avoids skin compression, which produces below normal scores. Take duplicate measurements at each site and average the scores. Usually six common anatomic landmarks are taken into consideration for anthropometric measurement:

- Right upper arm (biceps): Arm remains straight and extended in front of the body; measurement is taken at the midpoint between the shoulder and the elbow.
- Right forearm: Maximum girth with arm extended in front of the body.
- Abdomen: 1 inch above the umbilicus.
- Buttocks: Maximum protrusion with heels together.

- Right thigh: Upper thigh, just below the buttocks.
- Right calf: Widest girth midway between ankle and knee.

Different prediction equations based on girths exist for each gender and various age groups (McArdle et al. 2001). The equations for these subgroups, although cross-validated on different samples with moderate validity, nevertheless show significant population specifically. The equations do not apply to individuals who (i) appear overly thin or excessively fat, (ii) train regularly in strenuous endurance sports or activities with a substantial resistance-training component, and (iii) differ in race from the specific group used to derive the original equations (Brandon and Boileau, 1992).

Usefulness of Girth Scores

Girth is proved to be the most useful in ranking individuals within a group according to relative fatness. As with skinfolds, girth-based equations can predict body density and/or percentage body fat. The equations and constants presented in 'body composition' on the LWW.

Bioelectrical Impedance Analysis (BIA)

The measurement of human body composition by bioelectrical impedance analysis assumes that the body consists of two compartments—(i) the fat-free mass and (ii) fat mass. The fat-free mass contains virtually all the electrolytes and body fluids which are involved in conduction, so that the impedance of the body can be used as an estimate of fat-free mass. In this method, a small alternating current flowing between two electrodes passes through hydrated fat-free body tissues and extracellular water more rapidly than fat or bony tissues. It occurs because of the greater electrolyte content (lower electrical resistance) of the fat-free component (Figs 14.6A and B).

The impedance of a conductor is related to its length and cross-sectional area:

$z = rL/A$

Where, z is the impedance in Ohms, r is the volume resistivity in Ohm- cm, L is the length of the conductor in cm, A is the area in square centimeters.

Multiplying L/L gives $z = rL^{2/AL}$

Where, AL will be equal to the volume V^4

$z = rL^2/V^4$

$V^4 = rL^2/z$

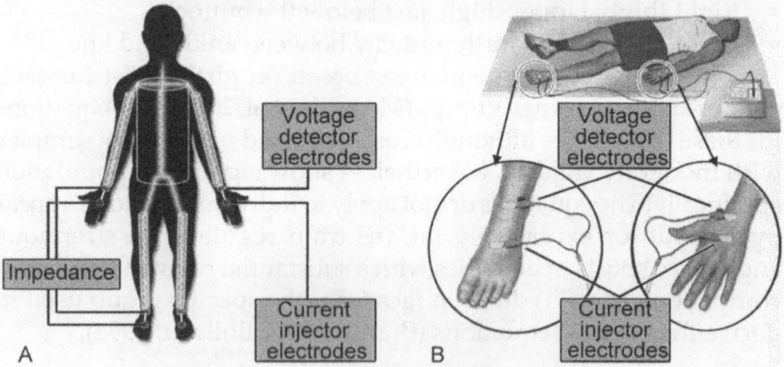

Figs 14.6A and B: Bioelectrical impedance analysis

Bioelectrical impedance was not used in the evaluation of human body composition until 1981 when Nyboer developed a tetrapolar electrode method. Four electrodes placed on the dorsal surfaces of the hands and feet are used to minimize the contact impedance. A current of 800 μA at 50 KHz is applied at the distal electrodes, and the voltage drop at the proximal electrodes is measured. The operator should be aware of the displacement of the electrodes by 1cm at wrist and ankle will produce a combined change in impedance of 4.1%, equivalent to a 3% change in body mass as fat.

As the technique is dependent upon the water content of the body, factors which may alter body water content, such as alcohol consumption and exercise before measurement are avoided. Either dehydration or overhydration affects the normal concentration of electrolytes in the body. This affects the current flow, in consequences, independent of real body composition changes. More specifically a loss of water will decrease the impedance measurement to yield a low fat percentage, whereas overhydration will produce the opposite effect. Skin temperature which is influenced by ambient conditions, also affects whole body resistance and thus the prediction of body fat by BIA. Predicted body fat is significantly lower in a warm environment (moist skin produces less impedance to electrical flow) as compared to cold one (Carton et al. 1987).

Method: A person lies on a flat, nonconducting surface, with injector (source) electrodes attached on the dorsal surface of the foot and wrist. Skin is firmly scrubbed with the help of surgical spirit over the areas where the sensor pads are to be placed ensuring that the skin is completely dry. This procedure removes all dead skin and excess oils that prevent good contact with sensor pads.

On the hand, sensor pads are centrally directed above the third knuckle of the middle finger. Second sensor pad is placed on the crease of the wrist where the hand is bent back. The sensor pads on the foot are centrally directed where the second and third toe meet the foot. Second pad is placed at the crease of the ankle in line with the shin bone.

Cable connection: On hand using either of the two main wires, clip the negative (black) to the sensor pads on the knuckle and the positive (red) to the pad on the wrist. On foot, clip the negative (black) to the pad nearer to the toes and the positive (red) to the pad on the ankle for testing.

The body of the person should be completely relaxed. Legs and hands should not be bent or crossed. Hands, palms should be flat on the side, away from the body, legs flat and slightly apart.

To obtain the measurements, tune on the bioelectrical impedance analysis pressing ON/OFF button once. To select 'Metric/Imperial' reading press 'PROG' key once. The display show (lmperial) = l. M (Metric) = 0. Select the unit and 'ENTER'. Sex, height, weight and age are entered. The display now shows processing for 10 seconds. 'BLEEP' indicates the test has been completed. Required readings are obtained by pressing suitable keys.

Drawbacks: It is found that even with normal hydration and environmental temperature, the prediction of body fat with BIA is less satisfactory than hydrostatic weighing. Lukashi (1993) was of the opinion that BIA tends to over predict body fat in lean and athletic subjects and under predict body fat in obese subjects. The tendency to overestimate true percentage body fat may be more pronounced among black athletes.

At best, BIA represents another noninvasive, safe, relatively easy, and reliable means to assess total body water. The BIA technique requires that experienced persons make measurements under strictly standardized conditions, particularly electrode placement and the subject's body position, hydration status, plasma osmolarity and sodium concentration, previous food and beverage intake, skin temperature and recent physical activity. Level of body fatness and racial characteristics probably also influence BIA's predictive accuracy. With proper measurement standardization, the menstrual cycle does not affect body composition assessment by BIA.

Near-Infrared Interactance Light Technology

This method is based on the principle of light absorption and reflection. A fiber-optic probe is positioned over the belly of the biceps muscle of the arm and an infrared light beam is emitted. Reflected energy or light absorption is monitored as the light beam penetrates subcutaneous fat and muscle and is reflected off the bone and conducted to the optical detector in the probe. All organic materials (i.e. fat or protein) absorb light in unique portions of the spectrum. The Futrex-5000 emits near infrared light at very precise frequencies (938 mm and 998 mm) into your body-frequency at which your body fat absorb the light and your lean body mass reflects the light. In essence, we are measuring how much light is emitted from the light wand and how much light is reflected back into the light wand. This measurement provides an estimation of the distribution between your body fat and your lean body mass.

The use of near-infrared light interaction to determine body composition was first investigated by Conway et at. (1991). They found that near-infrared spectral data from the biceps of the dominant arm alone resulted in correlation coefficients equal to underwater weighing values.

The measurement is taken at the midpoint of the dominant biceps. Years of research of US. Department of Agriculture have shown that taking measurements at all of the anatomical sites that are recommended with skinfold caliper will not significantly improve the accuracy of the technology. Even, though men carry most of their body fat in their abdomen area and women carry most of their fat in their thigh region, measurements taken solely in these regions would significantly overestimate total body fatness because they tend to be the highest concentrations of fat in the body and therefore are not representative of the entire body. As body fat is gained or lost, the distribution of fat/lean mass will change at the midpoint of the biceps based on the premise that you cannot gain or lose fat in site specific area that is gained or lost throughout the body. Conway et al. (1991) opined that the combination of skin thickness and subcutaneous fat thickness at the biceps allowed for optimal penetration and interactance of the low level of infrared radiation.

Arm X-ray Method

The arm radiograph is a useful method for analysis of body composition that permits quantification of reliable and valid estimates of body fat. The objective of the X-ray assessment is to provide a direct and unambiguous estimate of body fat content. The thickness of body fat layers at different points is transformed into a value of body fat for the individual by use of the fat fold surface area equation. The only difference is that, the fat thickness from the roentgenogram is substituted for fat folds and the K constant is derived in the same manner and differs among individuals depending on age, level of fitness assessed by VO_2 max and race. The validity of the X-ray procedure was determined by comparing values of fatness based on the roentgenogram and densitometry. The relationship between the two methods of estimating body fat was high (correlation on r = ~0.90 in young and older White and Black men and women). For an individual, the conversion of the X-ray widths of fat to total body fat percentage was accurate within ±3% units of body fat determined by hydrostatically. This degree of accuracy is generally higher than for estimates of body fat derived from fat folds or girths. The application of the X-ray procedure also include assessment of muscle hypertrophy that is useful in cross-sectional and longitudinal studies of body composition and aging, as well as chemical evaluations of nutritional status.

Ultrasound Assessment of Fat

With the help of ultrasound technology one can assess the thickness of different tissues (fat and muscle) and obtain an image of the deeper tissues such as a muscle's cross-sectional area. The basic idea of the ultrasound method is to convert electrical energy through a probe into high frequency (pulsed) sound waves that penetrate the skin surface into the underlying tissues. The sound waves pass through adipose tissue and penetrate the muscle layer. After reflection from a bony surface they then reflect from the fat muscle to produce an echo, which returns to a receiver within the probe. In the simplest type of ultrasound (A-mode),the time required for sound wave transmission through the tissues and back to the transducer converts to a distance score to indicate fat or muscle thickness. It does not produce any image of the underlying tissues. In more expensive and technically demanding B-mode ultrasound, a two-dimensional image provides considerable detail and tissue differentiation.

Ultrasound exhibits high reliability for repeated measurements of subcutaneous fat thickness at multiple sites of an individual in the lying and standing positions on the same day and different days. According to Abe et al. (2002) the technique has application for determining total and segmental subcutaneous adipose tissue volume. It may prove useful particularly in the obese people who show considerable variation and compression of subcutaneous body fat with skinfold measure.

Ultrasound method is helpful to map muscle and fat thickness at different body regions. It can quantify changes in the topographic fat patterns and serve as a valuable adjunct to body composition assessment. Ultrasonic fat and muscle thickness determinations aid in nutritional assessment during weight loss or gain in hospitalized patients. In assessing tissue growth and development, structure and function of the heart and other organ, ultrasonic imaging serves as a useful clinical tool.

Computed Tomography (CT)

Computed Tomography provides detailed cross-sectional, two-dimensional radiographic images of different body segments when an X-ray beam (ionizing radiation) passes through tissues of different densities. Through the use of appropriate computer software, pictorial and quantitative information can be obtained from the CT scan in the areas of total tissue, total fat and muscle, thickness and volume of tissues in an organ. Research findings demonstrated the efficacy of CT scans to establish the relationship between simple anthropometric measurements (skinfolds and girths) at the abdomen and total adipose tissue volume measured from single or multiple pictorial 'slices' through the mid-thigh region. Despres et al. (1991) found in a Canadian cohort of 110 men that CT scans determined deep and total abdominal adipose tissue accumulation at the L4-L5 region; measures also include skinfold thickness and waist girth. It has been noted that the single cut through the L4-L5 region minimizes radiation dose and provides the best view of visceral and subcutaneous fat. A high correlation ($r = 0.82$) has been established between waist girth and deep visceral adipose tissue (VAT) area. In fact, men with larger waist girth also possess greater VAT. An increased amount of deep abdominal adipose tissue is associated with the increased risk for type 2 diabetes mellitus, blood lipid profile disorders, hypertension, and cardiovascular disease.

Magnetic Resonance Imaging (MRI)

Magnetic Resonance Imaging is a valuable, noninvasive means to gather information about the tissue compartments of the body. In presence of strong magnetic field, an electromagnetic radiation (not ionizing radiation as in CT scans) excites the hydrogen nuclei of the body's water and lipid molecules. The nuclei then project detectable signal and under computer control it rearranges to visually represent the various body tissues. It can be used to assess changes in a muscle's lean and fat components following resistance-exercise training or during different stages of growth and aging. It has wide acceptance for medical diagnosis such as muscular dystrophy.

MANIPULATION OF BODY COMPOSITION STATUS IN ATHLETES

Success is the main goal of all sports persons in any competition. For optimal performances, most athletes have the interest in optimizing their body composition for their respective sports events. Manipulation of size and body composition is quite frequent among sports persons, with the definite goal of increasing their chances of success in competitions. To get maximum muscle power and strength, athletes of specific sports try to develop excess muscle mass. Among footballers, players of various throwing events, etc. increments of absolute size, regardless to competition, are justifiable. Before competitions, during vigorous training session, some players loose weight. To get the desirable back, players go for getting extra mass. Even to maintain a constant body weight, the players usually do so. In body building, where projection of body musculature is the prime, athletes try to develop their muscle mass. Fogelholm (1994) states three major reasons for manipulation of size and body composition status in athletes:

1. Before competitions (boxing, weight lifting, wrestling, etc.) making of a specific body weight category is required.
2. During the competitions (gymnastics, distance running, skiing, pole vaults, etc.) athletes with light weight are thought to improve their performances.
3. During the competitions (dance, diving, figure skating, etc.) the lighter and leaner appearance of the athletes may influence the officials who do the scoring of their events.

Some times the strategies adapted by the athletes to alter their body mass and composition may put them at risk for various health problems. With the purpose of manipulating physique and body composition rapidly, athletes go for reducing energy intake, inducing dehydration or taking pharmacologic agents (e.g. drugs) which could have adverse effects on their health in the long run. Without not being certain about the effectiveness of prolonged manipulation of body mass and composition, athletes go for that and often call some other complications which affect their performance, normal body growth, hormonal secretion, resulting certain diseases. Knowingly or unknowingly, some over enthusiastic athletes take certain strength-stimulating drugs (which are banned nowadays) and become the victims of ill health in the later lives. The effects of manipulation of body mass and composition on the performance, physiology and health of the athletes are discussed in the later part of this chapter.

Weight Loss

Various methods are used by the athletes to reduce their body weight. Of these, balanced died and physical exercise programs are most common. Apart from these, restricted fluid intake, exercise- induced sweat, environmentally-induced sweating such as use of sauna bath and steam bath are also in practice (Fogelholm, 1994; Horswill, 1992; Walberg Rankin, 1995 and Weissinger et al. 1991). To a lesser extent, catharosis (forced vomiting and laxatives) and diuresis through drugs are also used by the athletes. Another obscure method sometimes used by the athletes is blood letting, in which a specific volume of blood is withdrawn and reinfused after the weight in (Buschschluter, 1977). All these methods of weight loss potentially affect the body composition, performance and physiology of the athletes. These effects are either acute or chronic.

Acute Effects

Body Composition/Nutritional Status

The immediate effect of weight loss on body composition is reductions in total body water and body glycogen stores. Research findings show the general trend percentage composition of daily weight loss during four weeks of dieting. Water makes up about 70% of the weight lost over the first week of energy deficit. In second and third weeks, the water loss is reduced to 20% of the weight lost. Houston et al. (1981) reported that in elite wrestlers who reduced weight by about 8% in three days reduced about 46% glycogen concentration in the vastus lateralis muscle. Tarnopolsky et al. (1996) supported the study showing about 54% reduction in glycogen concentration in the biceps brachii of wrestlers who lost about 5% of body weight. During four weeks of caloric restriction, body fat reduction was reported at 25% of the weight loss in first week, 75% in second and third week and 85% in the fourth week.

During acute weight loss in athletes, Walberg et al. (1988) suggested that an increase in fat oxidation and protein breakdown occurred. When daily protein intake is inadequate, the reduction of fat-free body mass occurs which may be related to negative nitrogen balance.

Performance

Rapid weight reduction in athletes is responsible for the reduction of muscle glycogen concentration (Houston et al. 1981 and Tarnoplsky et al. 1996). Inadequate glycogen concentration in muscles causes impairment in muscle ability to sustain contractions at a set workload for long-duration (Costill, 1988 and Costill and Hargreaves, 1992). Sewka et al. (1984) and Montain and Coyle (1992) stated that rapid weight loss along with dehydration, reduced plasma volume causing cardiac output and thermoregulatory capabilities which promote exertion. Therefore, rapid weight reduction adversely affects submaximal endurance performance, especially in aerobic metabolism. With repeated bouts, the muscle depends on external metabolic pathways and systems of recovery. Rapid weight loss often causes limited blood flow to muscle and skin resulting deprivation of nutrients and weakening heat dissipation and subsequently causing fatigue in the muscle. But in short duration, and single high power bouts of exertion, the rapid weight reduction has no effect (Horswill, 1993). The possible causes may be, the short duration of high intensity efforts require anaerobic metabolism on a prime source of production of energy. The muscles remain self- sufficient to perform at optimal levels. Moreover, reduced body weight requires less energy cost in performing anaerobic events.

Physiology/Metabolism

As mentioned earlier that rapid weight loss along with dehydration causes reduction in plasma volume. During sustained, moderate intensity exercise, the reduced plasma volume causes reduction in stroke volume and cardiac output.

Herbert and Ribisl (1972) reported in collegiate wrestlers that after short-term weight reductions, heart rate had been increased at submaximal work rate.

This response compensates for reduced plasma volume reported to occur in wrestlers (Vaccaro et al. 1976) and rowers (Burge et al. 1993). Montain and Coyle (1992) opined that with increasing degrees of dehydration, the increased heart rate is not sufficient to maintain cardiac output. This change in cardiovascular function is transient. Once the athletes rehydrated, the heart rate and stroke volume return to their earlier counts. However, it is not clear whether recovery may occur for all degrees of weight loss. In resting metabolic rate, a transient reduction of 17% was reported by Melby et al. (1990) in collegiate wrestlers who had reduced their body weight by about 7% during training session. It was also reported that fat-free body mass was reduced too, at the same time. Now the explanation becomes complex. It is extremely difficult that the reduction of resting metabolic rate is the acute effect of the food deprivation or a chronic effect of reduced fat-free body mass. After the training season, when fat-free body mass returns to the preseason value, the resting metabolic rate also increases and returns to the preseason rates.

Health Risks

With acute weight reduction, the most common health risk includes muscle cramps, heat exhaustion or heat stroke. Caldwell et al. (1984) opined that rapid weight loss along with dehydration increased the electromyogram activity which might be related to spasms and cramping of skeletal muscles. US Department of Health and Human Services reported that in 1997, three collegiate wrestlers died during the process of exercising to dehydration in inter-college competitions. The Centers for Disease Control and Prevention stated that the self-imposed heat stress combined with preexisting dehydration were the main factors for their tragic deaths. Croyle et al. (1979) reported in a scholastic wrestler that rapid weight loss caused pulmonary embolism. Earlier in another wrestler, McDermott et al. (1956) reported pancreatitis occurred with rehydration and refeeding. More researches are needed in this direction. Rapid weight reduction may adversely affect immune functions also. Kono et al. (1988) found reduced pathologic functions and stimulation of lymphocyte transformation in some female athletes who reduced about 3.7% body weight during a 2-week training period. In spite of the reduced stimulation, the values of the stimulation index remained higher after weight loss than controls. Though the serum concentrations of prealbumin and retinal binding protein index remained unchanged in the data of Kono et al. (1988), but decreased with sustained weight loss in athlete data reported by Costill and Sparks (1973) and Roemmich and Sinning (1996). Therefore, adverse effect of rapid weight reduction during intense training period is being suspected on the immune system of the athletes to defend against the viral infections during competition and thereafter.

Chronic Effects

Body Composition

Research findings suggest that with the chronic effects of rapid weight loss in wrestlers, percent body fat and total lean body mass decrease. These reductions depend greatly on major two factors. One is the method, viz. cross-sectional or longitudinal, and another is the models, viz. two component model or multicomponent model. In some cross-sectional studies, the consistency of these changes has been observed. Long-term longitudinal studies give accuracy of the reports. On the other hand, two-component model is subject to bias when certain assumptions are violated. The assumptions of normal hydration of the fat-free tissues of the athletes are often incorrect. Because athletes undergo weight reduction before each competition and recover to dehydrated state after competitions. The degree of these purposely manipulation of body weight is another concern.

Protein nutritional status of athletes is altered with the reduction of plasma proteins which are closely associated with the reduction of lean body mass. Horswill et al. (1990), in high school wrestlers who reduced their body weight by 6.6%, reported the decrease of retinal binding protein and prealbumin. Roemmich and Sinning (1996) recently reported 22% reduction in prealbumin concentration in high school wrestlers who had reduced their body weight by 7.4% during competitions. Speculations are there that due to rapid weight loss in young wrestlers and gymnasts, their linear growth stunts. The reasons may be behind these speculations are:

i. Effect of intense training when energy expenditure exceeds energy intake.
ii. Participants are purposely restricting their intake which may be considered as contributing factor not meeting their required energy needs (Theintz et al. 1989).

iii. Selection process, like short-statured persons are selected for gymnastic for their biomechanical advantages. Stature is again a multifactorial trait where genetics is one of the important factors, e.g. short-statured athletes, whose parents are also short, are selected for specific events.

Physiology/Metabolism

Though not much change in growth rate is reported in high school wrestlers, changes in plasma hormone concentrations have been found. Roemmich and Sinning (1997a) observed reductions in testosterone and insulin-like growth factor-1 (IGF-1) levels in athletes who had reduced body weight by 3.8% after long-term training. The decrease of insulin-like growth factor-1 was consistent with an increase in growth hormone levels, but the concentrations of insulin-like growth factor-1 binding protein-3 were unchanged.

Insulin-like growth factor-1 acts as growth hormone resistance factor, that is why with the reduction of IGF-1 levels increase the growth hormone levels and do not affect the individuals' linear growth rate. The decrease in IGF-1 may not have been sustained for a long enough periods to stunt growth rate. After the conclusion of the season of competition and weight loss, the IGF-1 returns to the baseline level. In spite of a large reduction in IGF-1 and the increase in growth hormone, the concentrations remain within the normal range. McMurray et al. (1991) documented reduction of IGF-1 levels after short-term weight loss in collegiate wrestlers. Strauss et al. (1985) compared the in-season values and post-season values of testosterone levels in collegiate wrestlers and found that in-season values were pathologically low. It has been established that testosterone levels have a close association with changes in parent body fat. Greater the decrease in percent body fat, lower the in-season values of testosterone. The findings of Bemben et al. (1997) indicate that collegiate wrestlers may have low testosterone levels before the competition and subsequent weight loss. Then controversy comes, whether over-training or weight loss is the prime controlling factor for the alteration of testosterone levels. Majority of longitudinal studies conducted over the course of the competition season found less evidence for changing in training intensity and length that might affect body composition and hormonal status. In fact, once athletes reach the point of perpetual competition events in the season, they often reduce the amount of resistance training. Such changes contribute to weight loss or the loss of lean body mass.

Endocrine Disorders

Due to intense training and weight loss, female athletes often suffer from endocrine disorders viz. amenorrhea, delayed menarche, etc. Malina et al. (1973 and 1978) reported that the athletes reached the menarche at a later age than nonathletes. The average age of menarche in nonathletes was reported at 12 to 15 years and in athletes at 13.5 to 15.5 years. For each year of training before menarche, there is a delay of about five months before the onset of menses (Frisch et al. 1981). In the findings of Kashyap et al. (2007), some work is done in this direction and the data are presented in Table 14.3.

Table 14.3: Age at menarche in sports women

Events		13 yrs	14 yrs	15 yrs	16 yrs	17 yrs	Total
Athletics	Abs. No	4	5	5	6	5	25
	%age	2.66	3.33	3.33	4.00	3.33	16.66
Volleyball	Abs. No	4	3	7	–	–	14
	%age	2.66	2.00	4.66	–	–	9.33
Handball	Abs. No	2	5	7	6	–	20
	%age	1.33	3.33	4.66	4.00	–	13.33
Gymnastics	Abs. No	3	7	4	1	–	15
	%age	2.00	4.66	2.66	0.66	–	10.00
Kho-kho	Abs. No	2	11	11	1	–	25
	%age	1.33	7.33	7.33	0.66	–	16.66
Hockey	Abs. No	–	7	5	2	–	14
	%age	–	4.66	3.33	1.33	–	9.33
Football	Abs. No	1	3	11	9	–	24
	%age	0.66	2.00	7.33	6.00	–	16.66
Kabaddi	Abs. No	–	4	8	–	–	12
	%age	–	2.66	5.33	–	–	8.00
Total	Abs. No	16	45	58	25	5	149
	%age	10.66	30.00	38.66	16.66	4.00	100.00

Amenorrhea is the cessation of menstrual period for three or more consecutive menstrual cycles after menarche. It is seen that the competitive training and subsequent weight loss affects the menstrual cycle. It precedes the loss of bone mineral content causing an increased susceptibility of stress fractures. The long-term implications of amenorrhea include osteoporosis later in life. Prevalence of amenorrhea in general population is found to be 2.5% and in athletes the range is from 3.4% to 66% (Shangold, 1988 and Otis, 1992). Oligomenorrhea is seen in more than 30% of athletes.

Duration of normal menstrual cycle is 21 to 35 days, with a luteal phase of 12 to 16 days dominated by progesterone effects on endometrium. Alteration in luteal phase length and progesterone secretion leads to anovulation. Studies show that intense exercise and low body fatness have an effect on the length of luteal phase. Shangold et al. (1979) demonstrated that length of luteal phase decreased with an increase in the running mileage. Bonen et al. (1981) in their study, compared teenage swimmers to a control group of teenagers and fertile adult women and found that athletes had a short luteal phase. Studies have shown that women with athletic amenorrhea present with a reduction in luteinizing hormone (LH) pulse frequencies (Loucks et al. 1989). Morris et al. (1999) demonstrated significant reduction in ovarian hormone function in athletes who trained the longest and lost great amount of body weight to achieve competition weight. The energy availability hypothesis provides the most widely accepted mechanism to date that explains the suppression of reproductive functions in amenorrheic athletes. Reports from Loucks and Heath (1994) support that LH pulsatility depends on the energy availability (dietary energy intake minus exercise energy expenditure) in women. There may exist a specific threshold whereby further negative energy balance signals the inhibition of hypothalamic GnRH neuronal activity. Loughin and Yen (1997) have shown that the hormone product leptin of obesity may play a role in reproductive status of female athletes. A diurnal pattern of 24 hours, leptin levels was present in normal cycling athletes and controls and was absent in amenorrheic athletes, further supporting the inter-relationship between energy and diet in reproductive system.

Osteoporosis occurs due to reduction of the mass of bone per unit of volume. The reduction is sufficient to interfere with the mechanical support function of bone and leads to increased incidence of fractures, especially of vertebral body, neck of femur, humerus and wrist. Factors leading to this condition in female athletes are hypoestrogenic state seen in exercise associated amenorrhea and reduced dietary calcium.

Bone density in both sexes, increases until 25 to 35 years of age. Lower bone age has been reported in young ballet dancers with delayed menarche and increased risk of stress fractures and scoliosis (Warren et al, 1986). Renckon et al. (1996) have demonstrated that extended periods of amenorrhea may result in low bone density at multiple skeletal sites (lumbar spine, femoral neck and shaft, trochanter, intertrochanteric region, ward's triangle and tibia), including those individuals who are subject to impact loading during exercise. Linnell et al. (1984) in their study, showed that amenorrhea independent of body composition, was not related to reduced bone mineral content in female runners, but the combination of excessive thinness and amenorrhea may predispose female athletes to lose bone mass. The same was found by Nelson et al. (1986) when they evaluated relationship of diet, exercise and menstrual status to bone mineral content of female athletes. They suggested that amenorrhea with abnormally low food intake had deleterious effect on the mineral content of trabecular bone. Drinkwater et al. (1986) demonstrated that reduction in training as well as increase in body weight preceded resumption of menses, which in turn lead to significant increase in bone mineral density of formerly amenorrheic athletes. Data from author's laboratory regarding menstrual disorders in sports women are presented in Table 14.4.

Although susceptibility for endocrine perturbations is mainly in female athletes, Hackney et al. (1988) reported that certain male athletes with reduced body weight might also be at risk. Wrestlers with reduced body weight have reduced testosterone levels. It is not clear whether reduction in muscle mass or bone mineral is responsible for these alterations.

Table 14.4: Menstrual disorders in sports women

Events		Amenorrhea	Oligomenorrhea	Dismenorrhea	Total
Athletics	Abs. No	–	2	18	20
	%age	–	2.04	18.36	20.40

Contd...

Contd...

Events		Amenorr-hea	Oligomenorr-hea	Dismenorrhea	Total
Volleyball	Abs. No	1	–	8	9
	%age	1.02	–	8.16	9.18
Handball	Abs. No	3	5	10	18
	%age	3.06	5.10	10.20	18.36
Gymnastics	Abs. No	2	–	12	14
	%age	2.04	–	12.24	14.28
Kho-kho	Abs. No	1	–	15	16
	%age	1.02	–	15.30	16.32
Hockey	Abs. No	–	1	2	3
	%age	–	1.02	2.04	3.06
Football	Abs. No	–	3	7	10
	%age	–	3.06	7.14	10.20
Kabaddi	Abs. No	–	–	8	8
	%age	–	–	8.16	8.16
Total	Abs. No	7	11	80	98
	%age	7.14	11.22	81.63	99.99

Performance

Numerous studies have followed up athletes to determine whether there is any importance of weight reduction on performance. Eckerson et al. (1994) and Roemmich and Sinning (1996) observed that the reductions in force production due to the weight loss, though some studies show no decrement (Freischlag, 1984 and Song and Cipriano, 1984). Reduced force production may be due to loss of fat-free body mass (Roemmich and Sinning, 1997) or decreased ability to recruit motor units (Eckerson et al. 1994). The findings of power performance are inconsistent may be because of the methods used. Body weight is the base of the resistance setting for testing anaerobic power. With the loss of body weight, resistance setting decreases masking reductions in power performances. It is also reported that mean and peak anaerobic power may be maintained after 4.5% weight loss in wrestlers using an isokinetic device (Park et al. 1990).

Weight Gain

Methods Commonly Practiced

Exercise and Diet

Attempts to reduce weight or to gain weight in athletes usually include changes in the training and diet. Specifically, resistance training to stimulate muscle hypertrophy and a diet adjustment to increase energy and protein intake are used. The extent to which muscle mass will increase is controlled by the genetic disposition of the individuals, but to some degree almost all individuals can expect an increase in muscle mass as a consequence of initiating a resistance training program.

Nutritional Supplements

Many athletes use dietary supplements to help increase muscle mass and strength for their performance. A perusal of any body building magazine will reveal an extensive list of compounds and supplements marketed with the claims of stimulating muscle growth. The explosion of numbers of compounds is in part due to changes in federal laws in late 1994. The Dietary Supplement Health Education Act (DSHEA) allowed the classification of non -FDA-approved compounds to be sold as dietary supplements rather than as food nutrients or pharmaceuticals agents. Restrictions on the claims being made also were relaxed relative to claims allowed for whole foods.

Protein and Amino Acid Supplements

Many athletes attempting to gain weight and strength will consume extra protein or amino acid supplements above the Recommended Dietary Allowances (RDA) in hopes that the supplements provide the structural components to synthesize additional body protein. Individual amino acids have also been consumed in supplemental amount in hopes that they will stimulate protein synthesis or inhibit protein breakdown by stimulating the secretion of growth hormone or insulin. In fact, resistance training may increase protein breakdown, but there appears to be a simultaneous stimulation of protein synthesis with the uptake of amino acids by the muscle cell (Biolo et al. 1995). Although the protein needs are increased over the RDA for both endurance athletes and strength trained athletes, few data suggest that increasing protein intake per se increases lean body mass and results in an increase in force production in well-trained athletes. For example, one study indicated that in healthy older man an increase in protein intake by 50% of the RDA combined with resistance training for 12 weeks resulted in a 139% increase in thigh muscle volume ($P < 0.05$) over that of the control group (exercise only) (Meredith et al. 1992). Both groups showed gains of similar magnitude (19-20 kg) for the one repetition maximum strength test, however. Others documented the greater increases in body mass (Meredith et al. 1992 and Fern et al. 1991), protein synthesis (Fern et al. 1991), and nitrogen balance (Lemon et al. 1992) with supplemental protein intake, but none of these studies tested the subjects for changes in strength.

Creatine

No doubt, creatine monohydrates are currently the most popular supplement on the market. Loading with doses of 25 g of creatine per day for a 5 to 7 day period followed by a maintenance phase of 2 g/day is pervasive in athletic circles. Initially, researchers are of opinion that, by loading muscle with this intermediate for carrying energy for high intensity performance, maximal force production could be enhanced (Greenhaff et al. 1998 and Harris et al. 1992).

The performance of repeated sprint intervals in laboratory experiments suggested that an attenuation of fatigue may occur in the later intervals after creatine loading. Findings for performance involving a single power effort or short sprint (12–30 seconds) and longer sprints (90–120 seconds) are less than promising for an ergogenic effect. The single study on endurance performance indicated a significantly slower time by about 26 seconds for a 6 km run open field running trial after loading with creatine (Balsom et al. 1993). The 0.9 kg average gain in body weight of the runners was suggested as the reason for the impaired performance compared with the placebo group, for which body weight and running time were unchanged after the treatment.

Secondary to the performance outcomes, a fairly consistent observation has been the increase in body mass of approximately 1 to 2 kg during the short, 5 day loading phase (Balsom et al. 1993 and 1995; Earnest et al. 1995 and Mujika et al. 1997). Supplement distributors claims that the increase is in the lean muscle tissue, with the implication that contractile protein mass has increased. Nonetheless, the rapid weight gain in such a short period has been coupled with a transient reduction in the volume of urine excreted.

This is highly suggestive of water retention, not an increase in cell protein mass. To this point, none of the short-term studies reporting an increase in fat-free mass have used research techniques that overcome the limitations of the two compartment analysis. A comparatively recent preliminary report confirmed that total body water and intercellular fluid volume were expanded after 3 days of creatine loading (Ziegenfuss et al. 1997). The study used BIS, which is still in the early stages of being validated for measuring acute alternations in the various compartments that compose the total body water (Vandenberghe et al. 1997). Nevertheless, by using MRI the concomitant measures of thigh volume were supportive by revealing an expansion of the cross-sectional area for the muscle. Potentially, with prolonged creatine supplementation in combination with resistance training, an increase in lean body mass may occur; the true contribution of creatine to stimulating an increase in protein content remains to be determined (Boileau and Horswill, 2000). Apart from creatine, chromium supplement is also popular among athletes. The latest ergogenic ingredient arrived in the market in β-Hydroxy-β-methyl butyrate (βHβMB), having anabolic effect with the capacity of speedy recovery after intense resistance training.

Glossary

A

A-band: Areas of the resting sarcomere where actin and myosin filaments overlap.
Absorption: The uptake of the end products of digestion through the cell membranes of the digestive tract and into the blood and lymph circulation.
Acceleration: The rate of change of velocity measured in meters per second per second (m/s^2).
Acetylcholine (ACh): An ammonium derivative that is an excitatory neurotransmitter; stored in the vesicles of the synaptic knob it is secreted from nerve endings during an action potential.
Acetyl coenzyme A, acetyl-CoA: The key to the Krebs cycle and the oxidation of carbohydrates, fats and proteins; produced from the conversion of pyruvic acid.
Acid: A substance that donates a proton.
Actin: Thin protein filament of the muscle which combines with the myosin cross bridges to produce shortening tension.
Action potential: Changes in electrical activity across a nerve or muscle membrane.
Active transport: Energy requiring movement of material against concentration or electrical gradients, e.g. ionic pumps.
Actomyosin: Refers to the interaction of actin and myosin protein filaments during muscle contraction.
Acute: Rapid onset and short duration.
Adenosine diphosphate (ADP): A high-energy compound which combines with phosphate to form adenosine triphosphate.
Adenosine triphosphate (ATP): The major high-energy compound essential for cell energetic.
Adipose tissue: Tissue characterized by large fat storage.
Adolescence: Youth; period between puberty and maturity.
Adrenal glands: Glands lying on the upper surface of the kidneys; consist of an outer portion, the cortex, and an inner portion, the medulla.

Adrenaline: Secreted by the adrenal medulla that acts as a neurotransmitter and hormone for the sympathetic division of the autonomic nervous system; also known as epinephrine.
Aerobic capacity: Maximum amount of oxygen that can be consumed in unit time.
Aerobic metabolism: The oxygen – requiring breakdown of food substrates to synthesize adenosine triphosphate.
Afferent nerves: Nerves carrying information from the periphery of the body towards the central nervous system.
All-or-none law: A maximum response to an above-threshold stimulus; a below-threshold stimulus results in no response at all.
Ambient: Pertaining to the immediate surroundings, e.g. ambient temperature.
Amenorrhea: Absence or suppression of menstrual function.
Amino acids: Nitrogen containing substances that are the basic structures of protein.
Anabolism: Metabolic reactions leading to the synthesis of body substances.
Anaerobic: Having the ability to live in the absence of oxygen, opposite of aerobic.
Anthropometry: The science which deals with the measurement of the size, weight and proportions of the human body.
Antioxidants: Substances which retard the oxidative changes in fats and oils, e.g. tocopherols.
Arrhythmia: Disturbance of the regular rhythm of heartbeat.
Arterial: Pertaining to the arteries, e.g. arterial blood.
Arteries: Blood vessels carrying blood from the heart.
Arterioles: Small blood vessels controlling blood flow to the capillaries.
Arteriovenous oxygen difference: The difference in oxygen content between arterial and venous blood.
Atrophy: A wasting away of tissue.
Autonomic nervous system: A system of autonomic control of the internal environment consisting of two divisions: the largely inhibitory parasympathetic division, and the sympathetic, largely excitatory division.
Axon: The long conducting fiber of the neuron (nerve cell).

B

Basal metabolic rate: Refers to the minimal muscle activity and other basic functions necessary for life of an organism.
Beta-carotene: A fat-soluble plant pigment, which is precursor of vitamin A.

Beta-oxidation: ATP production from fatty acids that takes place in the mitochondria of the cells.
Blood: An alkaline suspension consisting of plasma, red cells (erythrocytes), white cells (leukocytes), platelets, proteins, electrolytes, hormones and glucose.
Blood pressure: Pressure in the arteries generated by contraction of the left ventricle; systolic (central) and diastolic (peripheral) pressures are measured with a mercury or electronic sphygmomanometer.
Body composition: Constituents of human body.
Body density: Mass per unit volume determined by dividing body weight of the water displaced.
Body mass: Total mass of the body.
Bohr effect: Greater dissociation of oxygen from hemoglobin in response to carbon dioxide in the blood.
Bone: One of the major components of human body composition.
Buffers: Substances that resist a change in hydrogen ion concentration.

C

Cardiac cycle: The sequence of events during a single heart beat.
Cardiac muscle: Involuntary striated muscle of the heart.
Cardiac output: whole body blood flow; the volume of blood pumped from the ventricle each minute; the product of heart rate and stroke volume.
Catabolism: Breakdown of complex chemical structures into simpler ones, often accompanied by release of energy.
Catecholamines: Neurotransmitters mainly adrenaline (epinephrine), noradrenaline, norepinephrine, and dopamine.
Cell: The basic units capable of independent life; comprising a nucleus and cytoplasm except in erythrocytes and bacteria.
Central nervous system: The system that consists of the brain and spinal cord which coordinates and controls the body's responses to internal and external stimuli.
Cerebrospinal fluid (CSF): Fluid bathing the central nervous system.
Cholesterol: Fat-like chemical found in all animal tissues.
Circulation: Continuous transport of blood and other fluids by the heart around the arteries, capillaries and veins.
Citric acid cycle: Alternative name for Krebs cycle.
Coenzyme: A helper needed by some enzymes to accomplish a biochemical change.
Collagen: Fibrous protein that makes up a large part of ligaments and tendons.
Collateral circulation: Development of secondary blood vessels that permit blood to bypass an obstruction in the primary vessel.

Concentration: The amount of a substance in a given volume.
Concentric muscle action: Shortening of muscle fibers generating force.

D

Dead space: Volume of the lung that does not take part in gas exchange.
Density: Ratio of mass to volume.
Depolarization: Reduction of the electrical change across the resting cell membrane.
Diastole: The relaxation and filling phase of the cardiac cycle.
Diastolic blood pressure: Representative of the resistance to blood flow in the peripheral vessels.
Dynamic contraction: Alternation of contracting and relaxing of muscles.
Dysmenorrhea: Painful menstruation.

E

Eccentric contraction: Muscle lengthening whilst generating force.
Efferent nerves: Nerves carrying impulses away from the central nervous system.
Electromyography: Study of the electrical activity of skeletal muscle.
Electron: A negatively charged particle that is a constituent of all atoms.
Endomysium: Connective tissue wrapped around individual muscle cells.
Endosteum: Tissue surrounding the medullary cavity of the bone.
Enzyme: Protein compound that speeds up a chemical reaction.
Epimysium: Sheath of connective tissue which holds the muscle fibers in bundles.
Epinephrine: Hormone produced by the adrenal gland which stimulates body structures that are not innervated by direct sympathetic fibers.
Ergometry: Measurement of work done.
Erythrocyte: Red blood cell.
Erythropoiesis: Red cell production in bone marrow.
Erythropoietin: Hormone produced in the kidney that stimulates erythrocyte production.
Extracellular fluid: Fluid that lies outside the cell membrane.

F

Fast twitch fibers: Muscle fibers with fast contractile characteristics and a low capacity to use oxygen that are used in short burst of activities.
Fat-free body mass: Body mass minus fat mass.
Fat: Any one of the organic food compounds which form the chief component of adipose tissue. Each one contains carbon, hydrogen and oxygen in definite combination.

Fatigue: Inability to response fully to a stimulus, or inability to maintain a desired energy output.
Fibrin: The basis of a blood clot; formed from the insoluble plasma protein.
Fick principle: Method of measuring cardiac output.
Filament: Long protein aggregates, as in the actin and myosin filaments of the sarcomere.
Fluid: Substance capable of flowing, e.g. gas, liquid, etc.
Forced expiratory volume: The volume of air that can be expired in 1 second following maximum inspiration.
Free fatty acid: Fatty acids that are carried in the blood and are not esterified to glycerol but combined with proteins in the albumin fraction.
Functional residual capacity: Residual volume plus vital capacity.

G

Gland: An organ that secretes a product which may be used internally, e.g. adrenaline, or externally, e.g. sweat.
Glucose: Blood sugar.
Glycerol: Compound composed of three atoms of carbon combined with three hydroxyl groups that combines with fatty acids to form fat.
Glycogen: A polysaccharide consisting of chains of glucose molecules, stored mainly in the liver and muscles.
Glycogenesis: Formation of glycogen from glucose.
Glycogenolysis: Breakdown of glycogen to glucose-6-phosphate.
Glycolysis: Metabolic breakdown of glycogen.

H

H-zone: The central area of the resting sarcomere occupied by myosin filaments alone.
Hemoglobin: A protein with four oxygen binding sites found in the erythrocytes. Carries oxygen and carbon dioxide and also acts as a buffer.
Homeostasis: Tendency of the internal environment of the body to resist change.
Hormone: The product of a gland of internal secretion.
Hydrogen ion: Positively charged hydrogen atom; a proton.
Hyperbaric oxygen: Oxygen at higher than atmospheric pressure.
Hypercapnia: Abnormally high level of carbon dioxide in the blood.
Hypercholesterolemia: Abnormally high level of cholesterol.
Hyperglycemia: Abnormally high level of glucose in the blood.
Hyperinsulinism: Excessive insulin excretion.
Hyperlipidemia: Excessive levels of lipids in the blood.
Hyperoxia: Enriched with oxygen.

Hyperplasia: Increase in the size of a tissue or organ due to an increase in the size of the constituent cells.
Hypertension: Abnormally high blood pressure.
Hypothermia: Lowered body temperature.
Hypoxia: Oxygen lack.

I

I-band: The outer areas of the resting sarcomere occupied by actin filaments alone.
Inspiratory capacity: Maximum volume of air that can be drawn into the lungs following normal expiration.
Insulin: Hormone produced by the islet cells of the pancreas.
Interstitial fluid: Fluid that bathes all tissues and supplies all nutrients; it is part of the extracellular fluid compartment of the body.
Intracellular fluid: Fluid that lies within the cell membrane.
Involuntary muscle: Smooth and cardiac muscle capable of generating their own intrinsic rhythm, but is under the control of the autonomic nervous system.
Ions: Electrically charged atoms and molecules.
Islets of Langerhans: Cells in the pancreas that produce insulin and glucagon.
Isokinetic contraction: Muscular contraction in which a muscle puts force against a variable resistance.
Isometric contraction: Muscular contraction in which a muscle creates force with no observable movement.
Isotonic contraction: Muscular contraction in which a muscle creates force against a constant resistance causing either shortening or lengthening movement.

K

Ketone: A product of carbohydrate metabolism which is acid in reaction.

L

Lacteal: An intestinal lymphatic containing chyle.
Lactic acid: The result of the reduction of pyruvic acid during anaerobic glycolysis.
Lean body mass: Body mass that does not include fat mass.
Lipid: Fat, triglycerides.
Low-density lipoprotein cholesterol: Compound consisting mainly of cholesterol thought to be involved in the development of atheroma and atherosclerosis.

Lymphatic system: Network of vessels that carry lymph from tissue interstices to the lymphatic ducts.

M

M-line: Line of M-filaments that provide structural for the myosin filaments.
Medulla oblongata: The part of the brainstem which is continuous with the spinal cord contains the nerve centers controlling respiratory and cardiovascular functions.
Menarche: Onset of regular menstruation.
Metabolic equivalent: A method of estimating the metabolic rate of varying activities.
Metabolic rate: The rate at which energy and heat are produced.
Metabolism: The breakdown of substrates to provide energy; it involves anabolism, the construction of large molecules from smaller ones that build and repair body tissues, and catabolism, the conversion of large molecules to smaller ones.
Mitochondria: Structures found in cell cytoplasm that contains the respiratory enzyme systems responsible for ATP formation.
Motor end-plate: The connecting point between a motor nerve and a skeletal muscle.
Motor unit: A nerve and its associated motor end-plates and skeletal muscle fibers.
Muscle: Tissue consisting of elongated cells capable of generating force.
Muscle cell: A single muscle fiber consisting of several myofibrils made up of myofilaments bound by the sarcolemma.
Muscle fiber types: There are three types: Type I, slow oxidative (SO); Type IIa, fast oxidative glycolytic (FOG); and Type IIb, fast glycolytic (FG).
Myocardial: To do with the myocardium, e.g. myocardial infection.
Myocardium: Muscular tissue of the heart.
Myofibrils: Active subunit of muscle contraction that is a subdivision of the muscle fiber embedded in sarcoplasm of a muscle fiber.
Myosin: Protein that forms the thick filaments of the myofibril involved in muscular contraction.

N

Noradrenaline: Hormone of the sympathetic nervous system that induces a constrictor effect in blood vessels; also known as norepinephrine.
Nucleic acid: Large organic molecule composed of repeating similar units, certain nitrogenous bases, sugars and phosphates.

Nucleus: Large almost spherical structure, bounded by a membrane, containing chromosome and other components necessary for cell division and transmission of inherited characters.
Nutrient: A substance essential for the growth, maintenance, function, and reproduction of a cell or organism.
Nutritional status: Health of a person as influenced by the quality of foods eaten and the ability of the body to utilize these foods to meet its needs.

O

Ossification: Formation of bone.
Oxidation: A reaction when oxygen is added or an electron removed; the opposite of reduction.
Oxyhemoglobin: The major form of oxygen carriage in the blood.
Oxyhemoglobin dissociation curve: The sigmoid curve indicating the relationship between the oxygen saturation of hemoglobin and partial pressure of oxygen.

P

Parasympathetic nervous system: Generally inhibitory division of the autonomic nervous system consisting of cholinergic nerves.
Partial pressure: Pressure exerted by one gas in a mixture of gases.
Passive transport: Movement of material by diffusion from an area of high concentration to an area of low concentration.
Peak oxygen uptake: Maximum amount of oxygen consumed without the appearance of the oxygen plateau.
Pericardium: Fibrous sac surrounding the heart.
Perichondrium: Membrane covering the surface of cartilage.
Perimysium: Connective tissue surrounding a muscle bundle or fasciculus.
Periosteum: A touch fibrous membrane surrounding a bone.
Phalanges: Plural of phalanx which refers to any bone of the finger or toe.
Precursor: A compound that can be used by the body to form an essential nutrient.
Protein: Any one of a number of complex organic compounds containing nitrogen in addition to carbon, hydrogen and oxygen.
Puberty: The age at which the reproductive organs become functional.
Pubis: One of the three bones of the pelvis.
Pulmonary: Pertaining to the lungs.
Pulmonary diffusion: Transfer of gases across the alveolar-capillary membrane.
Pulmonary ventilation: Movement of air into, and expired gases out of, the lungs.

R

Receptors: Specialized cells that respond to specific stimuli, e.g. chemoreceptor – adrenergic, cholinergic, and mechanoreceptors— barorecepors.
Red blood cells: Erythrocyte; oxygen carrier of the blood.
Renal: Pertaining to the kidneys.
Renin: Hormone produced in the kidney that regulates arterial blood pressure.
Repolarization: Process of reforming the charged state across a membrane after depolarization has occurred.
Residual volume: Total lung capacity minus vital capacity; the volume of gas in the lung following maximal expiration.
Respiratory exchange ratio: The volume of carbon dioxide excreted by the lung divided by the volume of oxygen consumed: VCO_2/VO_2.
Respiratory quotient: The ratio of the volume of carbon dioxide produced to the volume of oxygen consumed at the cellular level.
Resting membrane potential: Electrical difference across the cell membrane at rest.
Roentgenogram: A photograph made by means of roentgen rays or X-rays.

S

Sarcolemma: Membrane of the muscle cell.
Sarcomere: The contractile unit of the myofibril.
Sarcoplasm: Protoplasm in the muscle cell.
Sarcoplasmic reticulum: Endoplasmic reticulum in the muscle cells that deals with calcium release, protein synthesis, glycogen metabolism.
Saturated fat: Fatty acid with the maximum number of hydrogen atoms.
Skeletal muscle: Muscle that attaches to the skeletal system and causes body movement by shortening or pulling action of muscle on its bony attachment.
Sliding filament theory: The process by which muscles fibers contract due to the interdigitation of the thick (myosin) and thin (actin) myofilaments.
Slow twitch fibers: Muscle fibers with slow contractile characteristics and high oxidative capacity associated with endurance type activities.
Smooth muscle: Involuntary unstriated muscle cell found in the blood vessels and bronchioles.
Sphygmomanometer: A device for measuring blood pressure.
Steroid: Substances derived from the male hormone, testosterone which has masculinizing properties.
Strength: Capacity of a muscle to exert force in one maximum effort.
Striated muscle: Characteristic appearance of skeletal and cardiac muscle fibers brought about by the arrangement of myofilaments in the sarcomere.

Stroke: Lack of oxygen to the brain caused by thrombosis or rupture of a blood vessel leading to some form of paralysis.
Stroke volume: Volume of blood pumped out by one beat of the heart.
Subcutaneous fat: Fat located beneath the skin.
Suprarenal gland: Alternative name of the adrenal gland.
Sympathetic nervous system: Generally excitatory division of the autonomic nervous system consisting of adrenergic nerves.
Synapse: The junction between nerve cells, and between nerve and muscle cells, where impulses are transmitted by secretion of neurotransmitters such as acetylcholine.
Systemic circulation: Circulatory system for the whole body with the exception of the vessels of the pulmonary circulation.
Systole: Contraction phase of the cardiac cycle when blood is ejected.

T

Tendon: A fibrous band of dense connective tissue by means of which a muscle is attached to a bone or other structure.
Testosterone: Male sex hormone having masculinizing properties.
Thick filament: The myosin fiber of the sarcomere.
Thin filament: The actin fiber of the sarcomere.
Thoracic: Pertaining to the thorax.
Tidal volume: The volume of air inspired in a single breadth.
Total lung capacity: Vital capacity plus residual volume.
Triglycerides: Three fatty acids on a glycerol molecule.
Tropomyosin: Protein in the muscle associated with muscular contraction by producing an inhibiting effect upon actin, myosin interaction.
Troponin: Protein in the muscle associated with muscle contraction by producing a calcium interaction that releases the inhibition on actin, myosin interaction.

U

Unsaturated fat: Fatty acid capable of accepting more hydrogen atoms.

V

Vagus nerve: A key nerve of the parasympathetic nervous system affecting the heart and respiratory and digestive systems.
Vascular: To do with blood vessel.
Vasoconstriction: Narrowing of a blood vessel.
Vasodilatation: Widening of a blood vessel.
Vasomotor activity: Principal means of blood pressure regulation.
Vein: Vessel carrying blood back to the heart.

Venous: Pertaining to blood circulating in the veins.
Ventilatory threshold: The point at which the relationship between oxygen consumption, or power, and lung ventilation increases sharply.
Ventricles: The two larger contractile chambers of the heart.
Ventricular fibrillation: Electrical activity of the ventricles that is rapid and uncoordinated, resulting in no cardiac output.
Venule: Small vein draining the capillary bed.
Viscosity: Resistance to flow of a fluid.
Vital capacity: Maximum amount of air forced to be expired after a maximum inspiration.
Vitamin: Organic compound occurring in minute amounts in foods and essential for numerous metabolic reactions.
Voluntary muscle: Striated skeletal muscle controlled by the motor center.

W

Weight: Force of gravity acting on a body, measured in newtons.
Work: Product of the application of a force through a distance.

Z

Z-line: A protein mesh that forms the limit of the sarcomere and to which the actin filaments are attached.

Bibliography

1. Abe M, Herzog ED, Yamazaki S, Straume M, Tei H, Sakaki Y, Menaker M, Block GD. Circadian rhythms in isolated brain regions. J Neurosci. 2002;22:350–6.
2. Ahlborg G, Felig P. Lactate and glucose exchange across the forearm, legs and splanchnic bed during and after prolonged leg exercise. J Clin Invest. 1982;69:45–54.
3. Ahlborg G, Felig P, Wahren J. Splanchnic and peripheral glucose and lactate metabolism during and after prolonged arm exercise. J Clin Invest. 1986;77:690–9.
4. Araujo-Vilar D, Osifo E, Kirk M. Influence of moderate physical exercise on insulin-mediated and noninsulin-mediated glucose uptake in healthy subjects. Metabolism. 1997;46:203–9.
5. Balsom PD, Ekblom B, Soderlund K, Hultman E. Creatine supplementation and dynamic high intensity intermittent exercise. Scand J Med Sci Sports.1993;3:143–9.
6. Balsom PD, Soderlund K, Sjodin B, Ekblom B. Skeletal muscle metabolism during short duration high intensity exercise: influence of creatine supplementation. Acta Physiol Scand. 1995;154:303–10.
7. Barwich D, Klett G, Eckert W, Weicker H. Exercise-induced lipolysis in patients with central Cushing's disease. Int J Sports Med. 1980;1:120–6.
8. Behnke HD. Uber Siebrohren-Plastiden und Pastidenfilamente der Caryophyllales Untersuchugen zum Feinbau und zur Verbreitung eines weiteren spezitischem Plastidentyps. Planta. 1969;89:275–83.
9. Bemben DA, Walker L, Bemben MG, Fetters N. Influence of preseason training on serum testosterone (T) levels in NCAAI Wrestlers (Abstract). Med Sci Sports Exercise. 1997;29:S218.
10. Berchtold P, Berger M, Cuppers HJ. Non-glucoregulatory hormones (T_4, T_3, rT_3, TSH and testosterone) during physical exercise in juvenile type diabetes. Horm Metab Res. 1978;10: 269–73.
11. Biolo G, Maggi SP Williams BD, Tipton KD, Wolfe RR. Increased rates of muscle protein turnover and amino acid transport after resistance exercise in humans. Am J Physiol. 1995;268:E514–E20.
12. Boileau RA, Horswill CA. Body composition in sports : measurement and application for weight loss and gain. In: Garett WE, Kirkendall

DT (Eds). Exercise and Sport Science. Lippincott Williams & Wilkins. 2000; 319–38.

13. Boileau RA, Lohman TG. The measurement of human physique and its effect on physical performance. Orthop Clin North Am. 1997;8:563–81.
14. Bonen A, Belcastro AN, Ling WY, Cordon GS. Profiles of selected hormones during menstrual cycles of teenage athletes. J Appl Physiol. 1981;50:545–51.
15. Bonen A, Belcastro AN, Ling WY, Simpson AA. Profiles of selected hormones during menstrual cycles of teenage athletes. J Appl Physiol. 1981;50:545–51.
16. Bonen A, Ling WY, MacIntyre KP. Effects of exercise on the serum concentrations of FSH, LH and progesterone, and estradiol. Eur J Appl Physiol.1979;42:15–23.
17. Boot AM, De-Ridder MAJ, Pols HAP, Krenning EP, De Muinck Keizer-Schrama, SMPF. Bone mineral density in children and adolescents relation to puberty, calcium intake and physical activity. J Clin Endocrinol Metab.1997;82:57–62.
18. Brandon LJ, Boileau RA. Influence of metabolic, mechanical and physique variables on middle distance running. J Sports Med Phys Fitness. 1992;32:1–9.
19. Brooks GA, Fahey TD, White TP. Exercise physiology: human bioenergetics and its application. Mountain View. CA: Mayfield Publishing. 1996;144–72.
20. Brown, C. and Wilmore, J. (1974). Effects of maximal resistance training on the strength and body composition of women athletes. Med Sci Sports. 6: 174.
21. Bullen BA, Skrinar GS, Beitins IZ. Endurance training effects on plasma hormonal responsiveness and sex hormone excretion. J Appl Physiol. 1984;56:1353–463.
22. Burge CM, Carey MF, Payne WR. Rowing performance, fluid balance and metabolic function following dehydration and rehydration. Med Sci Sports Exer.1993;25:1358–64.
23. Buschschuluter S. Games blood-letting. Swimming Technique.1997;13:99.
24. Caldwell JE, Ahonen E, Nousiainen U. Diuretic therapy, physical performance and neuromuscular function. Physician Sportsmed. 1984;12:73–85.
25. Carton N, Norem JK, Niedenthal PM, Longston CA, Prower AM. Life tasks, self- concept ideas, and cognitive strategies in a life transition. J Pers Soc Psychol. 1987;53:1178–91.
26. Christensen NJ, Galbo H, Hansen JF, Hesse B, Richter EA, Trap-Jensen J. Catecholamines and exercise. Diabetes. 1979;28:58–62.
27. Christophe J, Mayer J. Effect of exercise on glucose uptake in rats and men. J Appl Physiol. 1958;13:269 –72.

28. Conway DJ, Greenwood BM, McBride JS. Epidemiology of multiple-clone *Plasmodium falciparum* infections in Grambian patients. Parasitology.1991;103:1–6.
29. Cooper C, Cawley M, Bhalla A. Childhood growth, physical activity and peak bone mass in women. J Bone Miner Res. 1995;10:940–7.
30. Costill DJ, Hargreaves M. Carbohydrate nutrition and fatigue. Sports Med. 1992;13:86–92.
31. Costill DL. Carbohydrates for exercise: dietary demands for optimal performance. Int J Sports Med. 1988;9:1–18.
32. Costill DL, Sparks KE. Rapid fluid replacement following dehydration. J Appl Physiol. 1973;34:299–303.
33. Cowin SC, Moss-Salentyn L, Moss ML. Candidates for the mechanosensory system in bone. J Biochem Eng. 1991;113:191–7.
34. Coyle EF, Coggan AR, Hemmert MK, Ivy JL. Muscle glycogen utilization during prolonged strenuous exercise when fed carbohydrate. J Appl Physiol. 1986;61:165–72.
35. Croyle PH, Place RA, Hilgenberg AD. Massive pulmonary embolism in a high school wrestlers. JAMA. 1979;241:827–8.
36. Despres JP, Prud'homme D, Poutiot MC, Tremblay A, Bouchard C. Estimation of deep abdominal tissue accumulation from simple anthropometric measurements in man. Am J Clin Nutrition. 1991;54:471–7.
37. Drinkwater BL, Nilson K, Otts S, Chestnut CH. Bone mineral density after resumption of menses in amenorrheic athletes. JAMA. 1986;256:380–2.
38. Earnest CP, Snell PG, Rodriguez R, Almada AL, Mitchell TL. The effect of creatine monohydrate ingestion on anaerobic power indices, muscular strength and body composition. Acta Physiol Scand. 1995;153:207–9.
39. Eckerson JM, Housh DJ, Housh TJ, Johnson GO. Seasonal changes in body composition, strength and muscular power in high school wrestlers. Pediatr Exer Sci. 1994;6:39–52.
40. Elias AN, Wilson AF. Exercise and gonadal function. Hum Reprod. 1993;8:1747–61.
41. Fahey TD. Serum testosterone, body composition and strength of young adults. Med Sci Sports. 1976;8:31.
42. Fallo F. Renin-angiotensin-aldosterone system and physical exercise. J Sports Med Phys Fitness. 1993;33:306–12.
43. Farrell PA, Garthwaite TL, Gustafson AB. Plasma adrenocorticotropin and cortisol responses to submaximal and exhaustive exercise. J Appl Physiol. 1983;55:1441–4.
44. Felig P, Wahren J. Fuel homeostasis in exercise. N Engl J Med.1975;293:1078–84.

45. Fenn CE, Leipes JB, Light IM, Maughan KO. Effects of the oral administration of fluid, electrolytes and substrate on endurance capacity in man. J Physiol.1983;341:66.
46. Fern EB, Bielinski RN, Schutz Y. Effects of exaggerated amino acid and protein supply in man. Experientia.1991; 47:168–72.
47. Fogelholm M. Effects of body weight reduction on sports performance. Sports Med. 1994;18:249–67.
48. Forwood MR, Parker AW. Effects of exercise on bone growth: mechanical and physical properties studied in the rat. Clin Briomech. 1987;2:185–90.
49. Freischlag J. Weight loss, body composition and health of a high school wrestler. Physician Sports Med. 1984;12:121–6.
50. Frisch RE, Gotz Welbergen AV, McArthur JW. Delayed menarche and amenorrhoea of college athletes in relation to onset of training. JAMA. 1981;246:1559–63.
51. Frost HM. Skeletal structural adaptations to mechanical usage (SATMU). 1. Redefining Wolff's law: the bone modeling problem. Anat. Rec.1990;226:204–13.
52. Galbo H. Hormonal and Metabolic Adaptations to Exercise. New York: Georg Thieme Verlag. 1983;1-116.
53. Galbo H, Hummer L, Peterson IB. Thyroid and testicular hormonal responses to graded and prolonged exercise in men. Eur J Appl Physiol. 1977;36:101–6.
54. Galbo H, Kjaer M, Mikines KJ. Neurohormonal system. In: Skinner J, Corbin CB, Landers DM (Eds). Future Directions in Exercise and Sport Science Research. Champaign, IL: Human Kinetics Publishers. 1989;339–45.
55. Greenhaff PL, Casey A, Short AH, Harris R, Soderlund K, Hultman E. Influence of oral creatine supplementation of muscle torque during repeated bouts of maximal voluntary exercise in man. Clin Sci. 1998;84;565–71.
56. Gurr MI, Harwood JI. Lipid Biochemistry: An Introduction. 4th ed. New York:Chapman and Hall. 1991.
57. Gyntelberg F, Rennie MJ, Hickson RC, Holloszy JO. Effect on training on the response of plasma glucagons on exercise. J Appl Physiol. 1977;43:302–5.
58. Hackney AC. Endurance training and testosterone levels. Sports Med. 1996;8:117–27.
59. Hackney AC. The male reproductive system and endurance exercise. Med Sci Sports Exerc. 1996;28:180–9.
60. Hackney AC, Fahrner CL, Stupnicki R. Reproductive hormonal responses to maximal exercise in endurance trained men with low testosterone levels. Clin Exp Endocrinol Diabete. 1997;105:291–5.
61. Hackney AC, Sharp RL, Runyon W. Effects of intensive training on the prolactin response to submaximal exercise in males. J Iowa Acad Sci. 1989;96:52–3.

62. Hackney AC, Sinning WE, Bruot BC. Hypothalamic-pituitary-testicular axis function in endurance trained males. Int J Sports Med. 1990;11:298–303.
63. Hackney AC, Sinning WE, Bruot BC. Reproductive hormonal profiles of endurance trained and untrained males. Med Sci Sports Exer. 1988; 20:60–5.
64. Harris R, Soderlund K, Hultman E. Elevation of creatine in resting and exercise muscle of normal subjects by creatine supplementation. Clin Sci. 1992;83:367–74.
65. Hartley LH, Mason JW, Hogan RP. Multiple hormonal responses to graded exercise in relation to physical training. J Appl Physiol. 1972;33:1602–6.
66. Hawley JA, Schabort EJ, Noakes TD, Dennis SC. Carbohydrate-loading and exercise performance: an update. Sports Med. 1972;24:73–81.
67. Heaney RP. Estrogen calcium interactions in the postmenopause : a quantitative description. Bone Miner. 1990;11: 67–84.
68. Hedges GA, Colby HD, Goodman RL. Clinical Endocrine Physiology. Philadelphia: WB Saunders. 1987.
69. Herbert WG, Ribisl PM. Effects of dehydration upon physical working capacity of wrestlers under competitive conditions. Res Q.1972;43:416–22.
70. Heymsfield SB, Wang ZM. Measurement of total body fat by underwater weighing: new insights and uses for old method. Nutrition. 1993;9(5):472–3.
71. Horswill C, Park S, Roemmich J. Changes in the protein nutritional status of adolescent wrestlers. Med Sci Sports Exer. 1990;22:599–604.
72. Horswill CA. Applied physiology of amateur wrestling. Sports Med. 1992;14:114–43.
73. Horswill CA. Weight loss and weight cycling in amateur wrestlers: implications for performance and resting metabolic rate. Int J Sport Nutr. 1993;3 : 245–60.
74. Houston ME, Marin DA, Green HJ, Thomson JA. The effect of rapid weight loss on physiological function in wrestlers. Physician, Sports, Med. (1981);9:73–8.
75. Jimenez C, Melin B, Koulmann N. Effects of various beverages on the hormones involved in energy metabolism during exercise in the heat in previously dehydrated subjects. Eur J Appl Physiol. 1997;76:504–9.
76. Johnston CC (Jr.), Slemenda CW. Determinants of peak bone mass. Osteoporosis Int. 1993;3(Suppl.1): S54–5.
77. Jurkowski JE, Jones NL, Walker WC. Ovarian hormonal responses to exercise. J Appl Physiol. 1978;44:109–14.
78. Kannus P, Haapasalo H, Sankelo M. Effect of starting age of physical activity on bone mass in the dominant arm of tennis and squash players. Ann Intern Med. 1995;123:27–31.

79. Karlsson J. Antioxidants and exercise. Champaign, IL: Human Kinetics.1990.
80. Kashyap K, Koley S, Sandhu JS. Female specific problems in inter-university level gymnasts. J Sports and Sports Sci. 2007;30: 5-13.
81. Keizer HA, Kuipers H, Hann J. Multiple hormonal responses to physical exercise in eumenorrheic trained and untrained women. Int J Sports Med. 1987;8:139–50.
82. Keizer HA, Rogol AD. Physical exercise and menstrual cycle alterations: what are the mechanisms? Sports Med. 1990;10:218–35.
83. Kinderman W, Schnabel A, Schmitt WM. Catecholamines, growth hormone, cortisol, insulin, and sex hormones in anaerobic and aerobic exercise. Eur J Appl Physiol.1982; 49:389–99.
84. Kjaer M, Secher NH, Bach FW. Hormonal, metabolic and cardiovascular responses to static exercise in man: influence of epidural anesthesia. Am J Physiol. 1991;261:E214–E220.
85. Koivisto VA, Yki-Jarvinen H. Effect of exercise on insulin binding and glucose transport in adipocytes of normal humans. J Appl Physiol. 1987;63:1319–23.
86. Kono I, Kitao H, Matsuda M, Haga S, Fukushima H, Kashiwagi H. Weight reduction in athletes may adversely affect the phagocytic function in monocytes. Physician Sports Med.1988;16:56–65.
87. Kotchen TA, Hartley LH, Rice TW, Mougey EH, Jones LG, Mason JW. Renin, norepinephrine, and epinephrine responses to graded exercise. J Appl Physiol. 1971;31:178–84.
88. Kreamer WJ. Endocrine response to resistance exercise. Med Sci Sports Exerc. 1988; 20:S152–S157.
89. Lanyon LE. The success and failure of the adaptive response to functional load-bearing in averting bone fracture. Bone. 1992;13;S17–S21.
90. Lavoie C, Ducros F, Bourque J. Glucose metabolism during exercise in man: the role of insulin and glucagons in the regulation of hepatic glucose production and glyconeogenesis. Can J Physiol Pharmacol. 1997;75:26–35.
91. Lemon P, Tarnopolsky M, MacDougall J, Atkinson S. Protein requirements and muscle mass/strength changes during intensive training in novice body builders. J Appl Physiol 1992;73:767–75.
92. Linnell SL, Stager JM, Blue PW. Bone mineral content and menstrual regularity in female runners. Med Sci Sports Exer. 1984;4 : 343–8.
93. Loucks AB, Heath EM. Dietary restriction reduces luteinizing hormones pulse frequency during working hours and increases LH pulse amplitude during sleep in young menstruating, women. J Clin Endocrinol Metabol. 1994;78:910–5.
94. Loucks AB, Mortola JF, Girton L. Alterations in the hypothalamic-pituitary-ovarian and the hypothalamic-pituitary-adrenal axis in athletic women. J Clin Endocrinol Metabol. 1989;68: 402–11.

95. Loughlin GA, Yen SSC. Hypoleptinemia in woman athletes: absence of a diurnal rhythm with amenorrhea. J Clin Endocrinol Metabol. 1997;82:318–21.
96. Lukashi HC. Soft tissue composition and bone mineral status: evaluation by dual-energy X-ray absorptiometry. J Nutr. 1993;123:438–43.
97. Lutter JM. History of women in sports: societal issues. Clin Sports Med. 1994;1:263–79.
98. Luyckx AS, Lefebvre PJ. Mechanisms involved in the exercise-induced increase in glucagons secretion in rats. Diabetes. 1974;23:81–93.
99. Malina RM, Hoper AB, Avent HH, Campbell DE. Age at menarche in athletes and non- athletes. Med Sci Sports. 1973;5:11–3.
100. Malina RM, Spinduso WW, Tati E, Baylor AM. Age at menarche and selected menstrual characteristics in athletes at different competitive levels and in different sports. Med Sci Sports. 1978;10:218–22.
101. McArdle WD, Katch FI, Katch VL. Exercise physiology. Lippincott:Williams & Wilkins. 2001;794–819.
102. McDermott WV, Bartlett MK, Culver PJ. Acute pancreatitis after prolonged fast and subsequent surfeit. N Engl J Med. 1956;254:379–80.
103. McMurray RG, Eubank TK, Hackney AC. Nocturnal hormone response to resistance exercise. Eur J Appl Physiol. 1995;72:121–6.
104. McMurray RG, Forsythe WA, Mar MH, Hardy CJ. Exercise intensity-related responses of beta-endorphin and catecholamines. Med Sci Sports Exerc. 1987;19:570–4.
105. McMurray RG, Proctor CR, Wilson WL. Effect of the caloric deficit and dietary manipulation on the aerobic and anaerobic exercise. Int J Sports Med. 1991;12:167–72.
106. Melby CL, Schmidt WD, Corrigen D. Resting metabolic rate in weight cycling collegiate wrestlers compared with physically active, non-cycling and control subjects. Am J Clin Nutr. 1990;52:409–14.
107. Melin B, Echache JP, Geelen G. Plasma AVP, neurophysin, rennin activity, and aldosterone during submaximal exercise performed until exhaustion in trained and untrained men. Eur J Appl Physiol. 1980;44:141–51.
108. Meredith CN, Frontera WR, O'Reilly KP, Evans WJ. Body composition in elderly men: effect of dietary modification during strength training. J Am Geriatr Soc. 1992;40:155–62.
109. Miller WJ, Sherman WM, Ivy JL. Effect of strength training on glucose tolerance and postglucose insulin response. Med Sci Sports Exerc.1984;16:539–43.
110. Montain SJ, Coyle EF. The influence of graded dehydration of hyperthermia and cardiovascular drift during exercise. J Appl Physiol. 1992;73:1340–50.

111. Morris FL, Naughton GA, Gibbs JL, Carlson JS, Wark JD. Prospective ten month exercise intervention in premenarcheal girls: positive effects on bone and lean mass. J Bone Miner Res. 1997;12: 1453–62.
112. Morris FL, Payne WR, Wark JD. Prospective decrease in progesterone concentrations in female light weight rowers during the competition season compared with the off season: a controlled study examining weight loss and intensive exercise. Br J Sports Med. 1999;33:417–22.
113. Mountain SJ, Laird JE, Latzka WA, Sawaka MN. Aldosterone and vasopressin responses in the heat: hydration level and exercise intensity effects. Med Sci Sports Exerc.1997;29:661–8.
114. Mujika I, Padilla S. Creatine supplementation as an ergogenic aid for sports performance in highly trained athletes; a critical review. Int J Sports Med. 1997;18: 491–6.
115. National Institute of Health Consensus Conference. Optimal calcium intake. NIH Consensus Development Panel on Optimal Calcium Intake. Clin Appl Nutr.1992;2: 39–44.
116. Nelson ME, Fisher FC, Castsos PD. Diet and bone status in amenorrheic runners. Am J Clin Nutr. 1986;43:910–6.
117. Nelson RC, Fahrney RA. Relationship between arm strength and speed of elbow flexion. Res Q. 1965;36:455.
118. Nelson RC, Jordan BS. Relationship between arm strength and speed in the horizontal adductive arm movement. Am Correct Ther J. 1969;23:82.
119. Ottis CL. Exercise associated amenorrhea. Clin Sports Med.1992;11:351.
120. Park SH, Roemmich JN, Horswill CA. A season of wrestling and weight loss by adolescent wrestlers:effect on anaerobic arm power. J Appl Sci Res. 1990;4:1–4.
121. Passelegue P, Robert A, Lac G. Salivary cortisol and testosterone variations during an official and simulated weight-lifting competition. Int J Sports Med. 1995;16:298–303.
122. Poehlman ET, Rosen CJ, Copeland KC. The influence of endurance training on insulin-like growth factor-I in older individuals. Metabolism. 1994;43:1401–5.
123. Raynaud J, Caperou A, Martineau JP. Intersubject variability in growth hormone time course during different types of work. J Appl Physiol.1983;55:1682–7.
124. Rebuffe-Scrive M, Bjorntorp P. Regional adipose tissue metabolism in man. In: Vague J et al. (Eds). Metabolic Complications of Human Obesities. Amsterdom:Elsevier. 1985;149–59.
125. Recker RR, Davies KM, Hinders SM, Heaney RP, Stegman MR, Kimmel DB. Bone gain in young adult women. JAMA. 1992;268:2403–8.
126. Renckon ML, Chestnut CM, Drinkwater BL. Bone density at multiple skeletal sites in amenorrheic athletes. JAMA. 1996;276:238–40.

127. Roemmich JN, Sinning WE. Sport seasonal changes in body composition, growth, power and strength of adolescent wrestlers. Int Sports Med. 1996;17:92–9.
128. Roemmich JN, Sinning WE. Weight loss and wrestling training:effects on nutrition, growth, maturation, body composition and strength. J Appl Physiol.1997a; 82:1751–9.
129. Roemmich JN, Sinning WE. Weight loss and wrestling training:effects on growth- related hormones. J Appl Physiol. 1997b;82:1760–4.
130. Rosenblatt JD, Yong D, Parry DJ. Satellite cell activity is required for hypertrophy of overloaded adult rat muscles. Muscle Nerve. 1994;17:608–13.
131. Ruiz JC, Mandel C, Garabedian M. Influence of spontaneous calcium intake and physical exercise on the vertebral and femoral bone mineral density of children and adolescents. J Bone Miner Res. 1995;10:675–82.
132. Shangold M, Mirkin G. Women and exercise. Philadelphia:FA Davis. 1988;129–45.
133. Shangold MM, Freeman R, Thysen B, Gatz M. The relationship between long-distance running, plasma progesterone and luteal phase length. Fertil Steril. 1979;31:130–3.
134. Shaver LG. Essentials of Exercise Physiology. Delhi:Surjeet Publications. 1981.
135. Slemenda CW, Miller JZ, Hui SL, Reister TK, Johnston C. Role of physical activity in the development of skeletal mass in children. J Bone Miner Res. 1991;6:1227–33.
136. Smith LE, Whitley JD. Relation between muscular force of a limb, under different starting conditions and speed of movement. Res Q. 1963;34:489.
137. Song TMK, Cipriano N. Effects of seasonal training on physical and physiological function on elite varsity wrestlers. J Sports Med. 1984;24:123–30.
138. Strauss RH, Lanese RR, Malarkey WB. Weight loss in amateur wrestlers and its effect on serum testosterone levels. JAMA. 1985;254:3337–8.
139. Sutton C, Tomkins G. Mechanisms of steroid resistance. Cell. 1974;2:221.
140. Sutton JR, Coleman MJ, Casey J. Androgen responses to physical exercise. Br Med J. 1973;1:520–2.
141. Tarnopolsky MA, Cipriano N, Woodcroft C. Effects of rapid weight loss and wrestling on muscle glycogen concentration. Clin J Sports Med. 1996;6:78–84.
142. Twin SL. Out of the bleachers. Old westhury, NY: The Feminist Press. 1979;XVI–XVII.
143. US Department of Health and Human Services (1998). Hyperthermia and dehydration related deaths-associated with intentional weight

loss in three collegiate wrestlers. North Carolina, Wisconsin and Michigan. Nov.–Dec., 1997. MMWR. 47:105–8.

144. Vaccaro P, Zauner CW, Cade JR. (11976). Changes in body weight, hematocrit and plasma protein concentration due to dehydration and rehydration in wrestlers. J Sports Med Phys Fitness. 16:45–53.
145. Vandenberghe K, Goris M, Van Hecke P, Van Leemputte M, Vangerven L, Hespel P. Long-term creatine intake is beneficial to muscle performance during resistance training. J Appl Physiol. 1997;83:2055–63.
146. Viru A. Plasma hormones and physical exercise. Int J Sports Med. 1992;13:201–9.
147. Walberg JL, Leidy MK, Sturgill DJ, Hinkle DE, Ritchey SL. Macronutrient content of a hypoenergy diet affects nitrogen retention and muscle function in weight-lifters. Int J Sports Med. 1988;9:261–6.
148. Walberg Rankin-JA. Review of nutritional practices and needs of body builder. J Strength Cond Res. 1995;9:116.
149. Wang ZM, Pierson RN, Heymsfield SB. The five-level model: a new approach to organizing body composition research. Am J Clin Nutr. 1992;56(1):19–28.
150. Warren MP, Brooks Gunn-J, Hamilton WG. Scoliosis and fractures in young ballet dancers: relation to delayed menarche and secondary amenorrhea. N Engl J Med. 1986;31:1348.
151. Weissinger E, Housh TJ, Johnson GO, Evans SA. Weight loss behaviour in high school wrestling:wrestler and parent perceptions. Pediatr Exerc Sci. 1991;3:64–73.
152. Welten DC, Kemper HCG, Post GB. Weight bearing activity during youth is a more important factor for peak bone mass than calcium intake. J Bone Miner Res. 1994;9: 1089–96.
153. Wilkerson JE, Horvath SM. Plasma testosterone during treadmill running. J Appl Physiol. 44:249–53.
154. Winder WW, Hickson RC, Hagberg JM. Training-induced changes in hormonal and metabolic responses to submaximal exercise. J Appl Physiol. 1979;46:766–71.
155. Wirth A, Holm G, Lindstedt G. Thyroid hormones and lipolysis in physically trained rats. Metabolism. 30:237–41.
156. Ziegenfuss TN, Lemon PWR, Rogers MR, Ross R, Yarasheski KE. Acute creatine ingestion:effects on muscle volume, anaerobic power, fluid volume and protein turnover (Abstract). Med Sci Sports Exerc. 1997;29:S127.

Useful Websites

- www.slideshare.net/LawrenceJames/histo-bone
- www.slideshare.net/LawrenceJames/histo-muscle

Index

Page numbers follwed by *f* refer to figure.